OXFORD MEDICAL PUBLICATIONS

Multiple sclerosis

THE FACTS

Ageing: the facts
(second edition)
Nicholas Coni, William
Davidson, and Stephen Webster

Allergy: the facts
Robert J. Davies and
Susan Oliver

**Arthritis and rheumatism:
the facts**
J. T. Scott

Asthma: the facts
(second edition)
Donald J. Lane and
Anthony Storr

Back pain: the facts
(second edition)
Malcolm Jayson

Bowel cancer: the facts
John M. A. Northover and
Joel D. Kettner

Breast cancer: the facts
(third edition)
Michael Baum (forthcoming)

Contraception: the facts
(second edition)
Peter Bromwich and
Tony Parsons

**Coronary heart disease:
the facts** (second edition)
Desmond Julian and
Claire Marley

Cystic fibrosis: the facts
(second edition)
Ann Harris and Maurice Super

Deafness: the facts
Andrew P. Freeland

Down syndrome: the facts
Mark Selikowitz

**Dyslexia and other learning
difficulties: the facts**
Mark Selikowitz

Eating disorders: the facts
(third edition) S. Abraham and
D. Llewellyn-Jones

Head injury: the facts
D. Gronwall, P. Wrightson, and
P. Waddell

Healthy skin: the facts
R. MacKie

Kidney disease: the facts
(second edition)
Stewart Cameron

**Liver disease and gallstones:
the facts**
A. G. Johnson and D. Triger

Lung cancer: the facts
(second edition)
Chris Williams

**Obsessive–compulsive disorder:
the facts**
Padmal de Silva and
Sidney Rachman

Parkinson's disease: the facts
(second edition)
Gerald Stern and Andrew Lees

Pre-eclampsia: the facts
Chris Redman and Isabel Walker

Thyroid disease: the facts
(second edition) R. I. S. Bayliss
and W. M. G. Tunbridge

Multiple sclerosis

THE FACTS
Third Edition

BRYAN MATTHEWS D.M., F.R.C.P.

Emeritus Professor of Clinical Neurology
University of Oxford

Oxford   New York   Tokyo
OXFORD UNIVERSITY PRESS
1993

Oxford University Press, Walton Street, Oxford OX2 6DP
Oxford New York Toronto
Delhi Bombay Calcutta Madras Karachi
Kuala Lumpur Singapore Hong Kong Tokyo
Nairobi Dar es Salaam Cape Town
Melbourne Auckland Madrid
and associated companies in
Berlin Ibadan

Oxford is a trade mark of Oxford University Press

Published in the United States
by Oxford University Press Inc., New York

First published 1978
First published as an Oxford University Press paperback with revisions 1980
Second edition 1985
Third edition 1993

A catalogue record for this book is available from the British Library

Library of Congress Cataloging in Publication Data
(Data available)

ISBN 0-19-262403-2 (h/b)
ISBN 0-19-262402-4 (p/b)

Typeset by Downdell, Oxford
Printed in Great Britain by
Biddles Ltd, Guildford & King's Lynn

Preface to the third edition

In the preface to the first edition of this book I expressed the fear that many of the facts about multiple sclerosis might prove to be unwelcome and disturbing to those who have the disease and to their relatives and friends. That this fear was unfounded has been shown by the many letters from readers expressing appreciation of an explanation of what is known and thought about MS. This I have tried to provide, steering, as far as possible, the narrow course between oversimplification and scientific complexity. This new edition is prompted by advances in knowledge, not, unfortunately, including effective treatment. I hope, however, that I have been able to show something of the great volume of research into many aspects of MS, and that this will be found encouraging for future prospects.

Oxford   W.B.M.

Contents

Plates

1 *What is multiple sclerosis?*

⁺Although there had been earlier partial descriptions, multiple sclerosis was first identified as a distinctive disease in 1868 by the great French neurologist Charcot, working at the hospital of the Salpêtrière in Paris. It may seem strange that a disease that now seems so well-defined should have remained so long unrecognized but methods of examining the patient with organic disease of the nervous system were only then being developed and Charcot's great contribution to medicine was in linking the careful observation of symptoms and signs of disease in life with the pathological findings in the nervous system after death. He called this new disease that he had separated from the many causes of paralysis to be found in the wards of the Salpêtrière, 'sclérose en plaques', a phrase that in his original lecture he feared would sound barbarous to his audience. The 'sclérose' or sclerosis of his title means hardening, and refers to the scarring that is the end result of the damage caused to the nervous system by multiple sclerosis. The word 'sclerosis' was used very freely in the early days of neurology and persists in the confusing title used in the USA to describe a quite different and much more serious disease of the nervous system, amyotrophic lateral sclerosis (ALS). The word is used elsewhere in medicine, notably in arteriosclerosis, or hardening of the arteries, which has nothing to do with multiple sclerosis. Another occasional source of confusion is with the word 'cirrhosis' usually applied to the liver and originally referring to the orange colour sometimes displayed by that organ when diseased. This again has no connection with multiple sclerosis.

The word 'plaque', still very much in use in the study of multiple sclerosis, literally means a tablet, that is to say, something with a flat surface. This is a misconception of the nature of the individual areas of damage to the nervous system—the lesions—and is derived from the appearance of such a lesion

cut across and viewed with the naked eye or through a microscope. As can be seen from Plate 7 this naturally presents a flat
surface—the plaque—but this is merely a cross-section of a
lesion that may extend a considerable distance through the
nervous system. In Great Britain the disease was originally
known as disseminated sclerosis, shortened to DS, a name that
emphasized an essential feature, that of *scattered* plaques
throughout the central nervous system. This name has gradually been replaced by that popular in America—multiple sclerosis
or MS. The main reason for the change was the existence of the
Multiple Sclerosis Society in America and the importance attached to ensuring that the Society in Great Britain was similarly
named. Disseminated and multiple sclerosis are the same
disease.

The nervous system

To understand the impact of MS it is necessary to have at least
an elementary knowledge of the anatomy of the nervous system
and of how it works. The central nervous system (CNS) consists
of the brain within the skull, and the spinal cord running down
the centre of the backbone. These are not, of course, separate
organs but join at the base of the skull. The CNS communicates
with the muscles and receives information from sensory organs
through the peripheral nervous system, that branches throughout the body. The distinction is important because the lesions of
MS are strictly confined to the CNS. The optic nerves that con-
nect the eyeballs to the brain are also part of the CNS and are
frequently affected in MS, but apart from this the plaques occur
in the brain and spinal cord only.

The CNS performs a great variety of functions, based essentially on the reception and analysis of information from the
outside world and from internal organs, and the initiation and
control of the response, whether this be movement, emotion, or
some more basic activity, such as sweating or evacuation of the
bladder. This crude statement should not be taken to imply that
the nervous system acts solely as an automatic machine, and

there is obviously much that is controversial or unknown, particularly with regard to such functions as consciousness, memory, and reason. All these functions, however, depend on the neurones or nerve cells, of which the nervous system contains some million million (a British billion) linked together in an orderly but literally inconceivably complex manner. Each neurone consists of a cell body and a variable number of elongated processes, of which the one that is of particular importance in MS is the axon. For it is along the axon, or nerve fibre, that the nervous impulse, generated in the cell body, passes on its way to link with other neurones in the nervous system or, via the peripheral nervous system, to effector organs such as muscles or secretory glands. The impulse, which involves both electrical and chemical changes, travels at different speeds according to the diameter of the axon in cross section, conduction being fastest in the largest fibres. To give an idea of the scale, the diameter of the largest fibres is of the order of one fiftieth of a millimetre. These large axons, and also many of those of smaller diameter, are surrounded by a sheath of a complex chemical containing protein and lipid or fat, and known as myelin. This is laid down in a spiral manner around the length of the axon (Plate 1) but is not continuous, being interrupted every millimetre or so by a short bare segment of axon known as the node. The myelin, although a chemical, is laid down and supported within a living cell. These are much easier to study in the peripheral nervous system and most of the experimental work has been done there. However, it is known that in the CNS it is a particular form of cell that is responsible for the myelin. The neuroglia or glial cells are the other major component of the CNS and are concerned with many supporting activities such as the nutrition of the neurones, and with the healing process. It is the group recognized under the rather formidable title of the oligodendrocytes (cells with few branches) that is responsible for the myelin sheath, each short segment between two nodes being formed and maintained by one oligodendrocyte. The functions of the myelin sheaths are not fully known. The comparison with an insulated electric wire, with the conducting axon in the centre surrounded by insulating myelin is certainly too simple, but it is known that myelin has an important role in accelerating conduction along the axon.

MS is often referred to as a primary demyelinating disease, by which is meant that the initial damage produced by the disease is to the myelin sheaths, leaving the axons intact. It is in fact difficult to be certain of the exact sequence of events in the formation of an MS plaque because the early stages are not often examined under the microscope. From studies of what seem to be early lesions, comparison with results in experimental animals that are probably relevant, and particularly from the study of magnetic resonance imaging (MRI; see Chapter 5) in MS some conclusions can be reached. As will be shown in later chapters, some of these facts are important when considering the cause of the disease and the means by which it produces symptoms.

Plaques

It now seems probable that the first event in the formation of a plaque is a breakdown in what is known as the blood–brain barrier. In the nervous system, in contrast to other organs, the cells lining the minute capillary blood vessels are closely applied to each other, forming tight junctions. This barrier gives some protection of the nervous system from changes in the chemical composition of the blood and also prevents the passage of white blood cells. The barrier is broken in many diseases and this certainly occurs in an acute MS plaque. Under the microscope, the earliest detectable change is the collection around a small vein of white blood cells—lymphocytes—that have apparently invaded the nervous system through the broken barrier. The lymphocytes spread along the course of the vein and are surrounded by an area in which the myelin sheaths have been destroyed (Plate 2). Opinion is still divided on whether the oligodendrocytes responsible for the formation and maintenance of myelin disappear from the early plaque, as these cells can be difficult to identify. It is not known whether the myelin breaks down because the oligodendrocytes are destroyed or whether the myelin, from whatever cause, is destroyed first. The plaque appears to spread by extension from the edges (Plate 3). The plaque and the surrounding tissues become swollen with excess fluid. The axons remain intact and can be seen running apparently undisturbed through the devastated area (Plates 4 and 5). As time passes the broken-down myelin is removed by scavenger cells and there is an increase in another form of neuroglia, the astrocytes, so called from their star-shaped appearance in stained sections under the microscope, and it is these cells that form the scarring or sclerosis. The lymphocytes disappear from the centre of the plaque but may persist at the edge where the disease process may still be active (Plate 3). In the chronic plaque it is still possible to see axons intact in the now scarred and otherwise burnt-out area but at this stage some of the axons finally degenerate and disappear.

The factor most likely to be responsible for the symptoms of MS does, therefore, seem to be the loss of myelin. There is experimental evidence to show that severe and extensive de-myelination completely blocks conduction through the bared axon. If the loss of myelin is less severe, conduction is slowed and, in particular, the transmission of a rapid series of impulses, of great importance to the normal functioning of the nervous system, becomes severely defective. That the axons remain intact is also potentially of great significance. If, within the CNS, axons are cut or degenerate from disease they may grow again from the end nearest the cell body, but the original connections are never re-established. This means that a disease that causes destruction of CNS axons is certain to leave permanent damage and, almost certainly, permanent symptoms. In the peripheral nervous system the chances of recovery are much greater, but even there the newly grown axons may not establish their original connections but go to different muscles altogether. Until a late state of MS, however, the axons remain normal in appearance and do not degenerate. This offers the hope that symptoms due to defective conduction in the demyelinated but persisting axons are at least potentially reversible in that they are not the result of irrevocable destruction.

As we shall see, spontaneous recovery from the early symptoms of MS is the rule but it is not obvious from examination of the plaques how this can come about. Authoritative statements were made that in MS the myelin could not be re-formed. This was surprising, as such remyelination is common in diseases quite distinct from MS that cause extensive demyelination in the peripheral nervous system, and is accompanied by recovery from severe paralysis. It has long been known that in some plaques the axons are surrounded by abnormally thin myelin sheaths, a few turns of the spiral instead of the normal thick sheath. This was interpreted as myelin in the course of destruction, but opinion has now veered strongly towards regarding these 'shadow plaques' as areas of remyelination in progress. If this is right, it could be one factor in the recovery from symptoms in a remission. It is, unfortunately, also plain that, at some stage, remyelination fails, as by the time they are examined most plaques are devoid of myelin. Another factor that is almost certainly important both in the production of symptoms and in the initial rapid recovery is the swelling in the plaque. The excess fluid could exert pressure on the bared axons and block conduction, which would be restored when the swelling subsided, even in the absence of myelin sheaths.

These then are the plaques. They are 'multiple' in the sense that certainly by the time the nervous system can be examined there are virtually always many plaques in different stages of development scattered throughout the CNS (Plates 6 and 7). It is not known whether the plaques are multiple from the onset of the disease, and in many patients the initial symptoms suggest that there is a single lesion. Even in advanced cases plaques do not seem to be scattered entirely at random. They are never completely symmetrical, but show a strong tendency to develop on both sides at certain apparently vulnerable sites, including the optic nerves and the spinal cord in the neck. The plaques are not only scattered in their anatomical positions but are also scattered in time, so that both the appearance of the CNS and the history of the illness indicate either successive outbreaks or, less commonly, continuous spread, often over 20 years or more.

The nature and pattern of MS

Apart from some inconstant abnormalities in the blood that will be described in later chapters, there is virtually nothing to suggest that MS is a generalized disease in the sense that tuberculosis, for example, can affect many different organs and systems of the body. MS does not affect the lungs, or heart, or skin, or even the peripheral nervous system, where the myelin has a different chemical composition. Whatever the final conclusion about the nature of the disease it is unlikely that symptoms are ever produced except directly or indirectly as the result of damage to the CNS.

This pattern of disease is not totally unfamiliar as there are obvious parallels with many diseases of the skin. Here, too, there is often no sign of general ill health and the colloquial word 'spots' indicates that the disease is patchy, with most of the skin free from blemish. Certain forms of urticaria, or nettle rash, and some rashes due to sensitivity to drugs bear a close resemblance to some of the features of MS. Particular areas of skin are involved, seemingly at random, while the rest is spared, although the noxious agent must be present throughout the body. The rash comes and goes, often with long intervals of freedom, and returns, often without a recognizable reason. Particularly striking is the rash known as a fixed drug eruption. Here, in response to a minute dose of a drug to which the patient's skin is sensitive or allergic, large round plaques of inflammation appear haphazardly about the body surface. These persist for a number of weeks, fading gradually, but if a second dose is taken they extend from the edges in a fresh ring. The capacity of the skin for healing exceeds that of the nervous system and no permanent harm ensues, even after repeated attacks, so the comparison must not be pursued too far. However, here is another disease, at first sight quite mysterious, producing multiple, disseminated plaques with intervals of recovery. Even in skin diseases where the course can so easily be followed, the cause may be difficult to uncover but once found, prevention is completely successful. There are certainly many enigmas in the disease process of MS but these are not the main obstacle to fruitful research as in many diseases effective treatment or prevention has been achieved without reaching the probably unattainable goal of total comprehension.

2 Who gets multiple sclerosis?

There are many strange facts concerning the distribution of MS in the world population that must be taken into account in any comprehensive theory of causation of the disease. Before describing these I must emphasize that all figures relating to the prevalence of MS must be approximate. Early cases are often not diagnosed because the symptoms have been slight or fleeting. The figures are also influenced in the opposite direction because, no matter how careful the examination, there are always some patients thought to have MS who are eventually found to have some quite different disease. Investigators are forced to classify their patients in separate categories of diagnostic certainty or doubt, the most usual being possible, probable, and definite cases, and other classifications are now coming into use. Bearing in mind these considerations imposed by difficulties in diagnosis the pattern of who gets MS and who does not can now be discussed.

The symptoms of MS are exceedingly rare in childhood. I have personally seen only two patients in whom the onset was definitely below the age of 10, and this is general experience. The frequency of onset of MS begins to increase around the age of 17 and reaches a peak in the early 30s. Thereafter the onset becomes increasingly uncommon but new cases, without any past history at all suggestive of earlier attacks, continue to occur into the 60s. Where notes are available, either from the hospital or from the general practitioner, it is astonishing how frequently people forget symptoms sufficiently severe to lead them to seek medical advice, so the age of onset of symptoms must again be an approximation. It is, however, quite well known that the diagnosis may be made only by finding a few scattered plaques at routine post-mortem examination in people who died in their 80s without apparently ever having experienced symptoms that could be attributed to MS. Indeed, it has been estimated that in Denmark, where a national register of people with MS is maintained, about one-half of those who actually have the disease never have recognizable symptoms. It is young adults and those of middle age who bear the brunt of the disease. In virtually every series reported, women are more frequently affected than men, the usual ratio being three women to two men.

There are two common methods of expressing the frequency with which a disease occurs in a given population. The annual incidence is the number of new cases recorded every year in some stated number, often 100 000, of the population. The prevalence is the number of people, again in every 100 000, known to have the disease on a given day. The former figure is obviously the one to use when dealing with acute short-lived diseases like influenza, while the prevalence rate is the more useful for most purposes in a chronic disease like MS. These figures are clearly partly dependent on the standard of medical care, the number of doctors capable of separating MS from other nervous diseases, and the accuracy with which the facts are collected and published. Over many parts of the world, for example, the Soviet Union, China, and South America, figures are scanty or non-existent. In many tropical countries, while no attempts at precision can be made, a fair idea of relative prevalence can be formed. Despite these deficiencies there is an impressive body of evidence from around the world for a striking pattern of distribution. The prevalence of MS varies markedly according to geography, and, with a few notable exceptions, the most obvious factor concerned is distance from the equator.

In tropical countries for which any estimate can be made MS is either extremely rare or does not occur at all in the indigenous population. In India occasional small series of patients have been reported, particularly among Parsis, but it is plain that general prevalence is low. In contrast, in north-west Europe and in the northern states of the United States of America and in Canada, in the northern hemisphere, and in southern Australia and New Zealand, prevalence is high, that is to say, above 40 per 100 000. In Great Britain the general prevalence is about 100 per 100 000 of the population, but even within these islands the figure is higher in northern latitudes. In north-eastern Scotland the prevalence is higher and in the Shetlands and Orkneys it may reach 300 per 100 000, the highest known prevalence in the world. Intermediate zones, such as the southern states of the United States, northern districts of Australia, and the Mediterranean shores have intermediate prevalence rates of from 20 to 39 per 100 000. If the effect was simply due to latitude the prevalence rate in Japan would be expected to resemble that in Great Britain, but MS is comparatively rare in Japan (though the severity is greater) and there are other anomalies showing that simple distance from the equator or some secondary effect of this, such as temperature, cannot be the only factor concerned. MS is, for example, said to be rare in Eskimos.

It is not easy to visualize the meaning of such figures in every day terms. One-hundred per 100 000 is 2 per 2000; one person with MS in a large village or in a single doctor's practice. Put like this the prevalence scarcely sounds 'high' but it has been calculated that in Ulster 1 in 1000 people born alive will develop MS. Odds of 1000 : 1 against are astronomical when it comes to backing horses but in densely populated areas they add up to a great many people with MS.

The figures from South Africa suggest that there is a racial effect on prevalence as MS occurs among the white population, although at a low rate, while it appears to be almost completely absent in the black population. In the United States, however, prevalence rates for white and black people, although still different, are much closer. These figures at first sight suggest that it is not race but geography that determines susceptibility but the relative rarity and increased severity of the disease in Japan remain something of an anomaly. There are also marked differences in prevalence between areas of similar latitude in America and Europe, being much higher in the latter. MS is not confined to those of European stock but there certainly appears to be a relationship between high prevalence and indigenous or colonizing Europeans, and some authorities have found this more obvious than the relationship to latitude.

There have been many detailed studies of the incidence of MS among restricted populations and particular regard has been paid to any hint that cases have formed 'clusters'. In virtually every study of this kind groups of cases have been found, apparently unrelated by blood or marriage but clustered in some small locality. The statistics used in working out the odds against clusters of a relatively uncommon condition occurring by chance are complex but apparently reliable. For anyone who believes that they have found some promising clues to MS because there are six cases in a small village it is disappointing to find how easily this could be a chance event. In those studies in which chance is statistically unlikely and some common environmental factor is looked for, nothing very convincing is found. In one survey MS is more common in rural areas, in another clusters occur in certain river valleys or on sheep farms but no convincing link between these different findings can be detected. For practical purposes, within a given area there are no consistent indications that any particular occupations or habitats are unduly hazardous with regard to the development of MS. The question of possible 'epidemics' of MS is discussed in Chapter 6.

A matter naturally of great concern to all patients with MS and their families is whether the disease is inherited. As will be seen in Chapter 6 on theories of causation there is evidence suggesting an inbuilt, genetically determined, factor that increases susceptibility. There is also increasing evidence that MS is more common among the close relatives of those with the disease than in the general population. Some studies have put the risk as high as 10 times greater among first degree relatives, that is to say, parents, brothers and sisters, and children. In one very careful study the chances of the child of someone with MS also getting the disease were found to be 100 to 1 against, really quite long odds. It is also clear that MS does not behave at all like any of the recognized patterns of inheritable disease. The science of genetics in man is a good deal less predictable than the results of artificially breeding varieties of peas, but nevertheless in many diseases, of which the best known are probably muscular dystrophy, haemophilia, and Huntington's chorea, the distinctive pattern of inheritance, recessive or dominant, can be detected and advice based on these findings can usefully be given to patients and their relatives. This is not so in MS and the findings from the study of identical twins indicate that the disease is certainly not transmitted by any form of direct inheritance. Identical twins, by definition have identical genes, and if one of these causes a disease both twins would be affected. Even in the most strongly genetically determined diseases the results are never quite 100 per cent, no doubt because factors in the environment also exert an influence. In MS, when one identical twin is affected, the chance of the other twin having MS is a good deal higher than in non-identical twins, and investigation may show signs of the disease even when there are no symptoms, confirming a genetic effect.

There is nothing that can be done about an increased risk in parents or in brothers and sisters, and practical advice must obviously be restricted to the question of possible transmission to children. In fact MS in parent and child is a good deal less common than MS in brothers and sisters. There have been claims that it is possible to detect by means of blood tests those relatives, in particular children of people known to have MS, who will develop the disease. These claims have never been substantiated and there is nothing to show that correct prophesies can be made or that there could be any benefit in giving any form of treatment to children said to be 'positive' in this test.

There may be other good reasons, medical or social, for a person with MS not to have a family or not to have a large family, but the risk of inheritance should not influence the decision.

Two separate studies in Great Britain have shown that MS is relatively more common in those of higher social and economic standing. Such figures are not easy to interpret but the National Health Service has ensured that these apparent differences cannot be due to better facilities for diagnosis being available for the comparatively wealthy. On a less scientific and entirely subjective plane many experienced neurologists have wondered whether there is not a type of person and personality particularly prone to MS. So often it seems to be the healthy, good-looking, stoical, and hardworking who are affected, people 'who put up with things better than one thinks one would oneself', as it has been expressed. This opinion may be quite erroneous but is one that has been strongly impressed on me over the years.

In conclusion, therefore, for practical purposes, MS does not occur in children or begin after the age of 55. It is commoner in women than in men, and in those with a higher standard of living. To be born and bred in the tropics is virtually to avoid all risk of MS. There is an increased risk of contracting the disease in relatives of those with MS but no clear pattern of inheritance can be detected.

3 *Early symptoms*

Before describing the common modes of onset I must refer to
a matter of great importance that caused me to have serious
doubts on the wisdom of writing a book explaining MS to the
general public. Following every surge of publicity I am asked
to see a number of people, usually young women, who are
convinced that they have MS. This is because certain of the early
symptoms of the disease that they may have heard described on
radio or television have a superficial resemblance to banal every
day experiences. To lie on an arm or to sit awkwardly with legs
crossed at the knee for too long causes temporary numbness,
pins and needles, and even weakness, as everyone is aware.
Many people do not have perfect balance between the movements of the two eyes so that, particularly when tired, vision
may become double for a moment as the eyes drift apart, clear-
ing at once after blinking or rubbing the eyes. Normally these
and other fleeting 'symptoms' are forgotten or rightly ignored
as of no importance. After perhaps listening to a friend describe
how MS began with numbness or double vision followed by
complete recovery it is natural to have misgivings about the
commonplace events I have described, even if only in moments
of anxiety or depression. Persistent fear, however, results in
other more persistent sensations; tingling induced by continu
ously breathing too rapidly, feelings of dizziness or uncertainty,
and doubts about whether knocking over the milk jug was
normal clumsiness or something worse. In fact these sensations,
by no means imaginary but certainly not in any way sinister, can
nearly always be distinguished from the early symptoms of MS
by any doctor with extensive experience of the disease, although
unfortunate mistakes are not unknown. To brood unnecessarily
and in secret is the worst possible way of coping. Fears are much
more easily dispelled if dealt with quickly.

As MS can affect any part of the CNS the initial symptoms can obviously be extremely varied. The distribution of plaques is not, however, completely haphazard and there are certain sites that are particularly vulnerable. In consequence the majority of the initial symptoms fall into well-defined groups.

Optic neuritis

As will be recalled, the optic nerves are part of the central, rather than the peripheral, nervous system and as such are susceptible to involvement in MS. In approximately 15 per cent of patients the initial symptom is what is known as optic or retrobulbar neuritis. These terms simply mean inflammation of the optic nerve and 'retrobulbar' indicates that this has affected the nerve some way behind the bulb of the eye—the eyeball. The original significance of these two labels was that in optic neuritis it is possible for the examining doctor, using an ophthalmoscope, actually to see the inflamed optic nerve, whereas in retrobulbar neuritis the inflammation does not reach the retina and the diagnosis can be made only from the symptoms. In a typical attack the vision is noticed to be blurred in one eye. It is not always easy to know how rapidly this comes on as, naturally enough, it is quite difficult to recognize even severe loss of vision in one eye if this does not occur suddenly. Some people only notice that there is something wrong when they accidentally rub the good eye while keeping the other open and are then startled to find that they cannot see clearly. The eye is somewhat painful (although not red or bloodshot) particularly on looking up or to one side, and vision continues to deteriorate for several days. The effect on eyesight varies from slight dimming of the normal vividness of colour appreciation to complete blindness in the affected eye, but the usual result is severe loss of central vision. This is most disturbing, as the act of looking at anything involves turning the eyes so that light from the object looked at falls on the area of the retina in which the light receptor cells are most densely packed. It is the axons carrying impulses from this area that most often lose their myelin sheaths in an attack of retrobulbar neuritis. These fibres do, in fact, make up a large part of the optic nerve, where they lie centrally and are therefore involved in any sizeable plaque within the nerve. Fortunately both eyes are rarely affected simultaneously.

Vision usually continues to decline for about a week but seldom for longer. At about this stage the pain subsides and a week or two later, in nearly every case, vision begins to improve. The expected result is complete recovery over the succeeding weeks with normal visual acuity as measured on the familiar wall charts. Sometimes, even when the lowest line can be read with ease, there may be a persistent awareness that vision is not perfect; colours may remain a little dull or contrasts of light and shade may be less sharp. Occasionally central vision remains more severely affected but even here there will have been great improvement over the initial loss of acuity.

This recovery is a characteristic example of that remarkable phenomenon in MS, the *remission*; a term that means substantial or complete recovery from the effects of an initial attack or subsequent relapse of the disease. It would be difficult to exaggerate the importance to the eventual understanding of MS of the potentiality for complete reversal of often severe disability. The implications will be discussed in later chapters.

There are other much less common causes of optic neuritis in which the nerve can be seen to be inflamed, but an unmistakable attack of retrobulbar neuritis is usually either found to be the initial episode of MS, or it may occur later in the course of the disease. The proportion of those presenting with optic neuritis who eventually develop other symptoms and signs of the disease increases with the length of time the patient is observed. Even with the longest follow up, however, there is always a number of people in whom optic neuritis remains an isolated event but at present there is no certain method of distinguishing this group at the onset.

Plaques in the spinal cord

The commonest site from which symptoms are produced during an initial attack is the spinal cord. Within the spinal cord run tracts or bundles of myelinated axons conveying nerve impulses to and from the brain and any of these may be involved in a plaque (Plate 6). Most frequently it is the tracts conveying impulses concerned with the brain's initiation and control of movement that are first affected. This bundle of axons is sometimes referred to as the pyramidal tract, a name that originates from the days of purely descriptive anatomy and refers to the supposedly pyramidal shape of the tract at a certain point in its long course from the cortex of the cerebral hemisphere to the lower end of the spinal cord. Many of the axons form connections with other neurones within the spinal cord whose axons in turn enter the peripheral nervous system and eventually supply the muscles. The effect of demyelination involving the pyramidal tract is weakness, nearly always of one or both legs.

The onset may be relatively rapid, particularly when influenced by fatigue. For example, the first few miles of a country walk may be accomplished normally, but weakness may make the return journey impossible. More usually, a weakness increases over a few days or a week or two, remains unchanged for a further few weeks and then recovers. The degree of weakness in a first attack is seldom severe and often amounts to dragging of one leg, inability to run and some difficulty on stairs.

The sensory tracts within the spinal cord carry nervous impulses derived directly or indirectly from a variety of sensory receptor organs. Sensations of touch, pain, and difference in temperature derived from the skin, and of pain from both the skin and internal organs are familiar enough, but there are other highly important sensory impulses that do not give rise to anything that we are normally aware of as 'sensation' at all. We are aware of the positions of our limbs, trunk, and head in space in a most precise manner without having to think about the matter. Information of which we are completely unconscious is fed into the CNS from minute structures in the muscles, ligaments, and joints sensitive to stretch. This sensory input is essential for the efficient control of movement and for many of the automatic or reflex reactions of the body to change of posture. The symptoms arising from demyelination in the sensory tracts ascending to the brain vary according to which of the different forms of sensation are affected.

A common mode of onset of MS is with a sensation of numb- ness in the feet, ascending in the course of a few days to the waist. Numbness implies loss of feeling, although it is often difficult to distinguish from loss of use, but it is seldom severe. A pinprick may still be felt as sharp but somehow distant. The loss of feeling may involve the bladder and bowels so that, although there is no loss of control, the normal sensation of passing water or of the desire to do so is absent. Vaginal sensation may also be absent or unpleasantly distorted. There is no difficulty in walking as neither strength nor the sensory inflow from the muscles and joints is affected. Remission normally occurs after several weeks.

These abnormal sensations are quite different from those experienced by people who have developed a fear of MS. They consist of vague tingling and numbness that moves about from one limb to another, or to the face, usually, for some reason, on the left side. They may be completely absent for a whole day or come on for an hour or two at any time, but are not constantly present. Such symptoms may naturally cause alarm but are not the symptoms of MS or of any serious disease.

Rather more disabling is an initial attack in which the sense of position, the knowledge of where the limb is in space, is lost. When this occurs it usually affects the upper limb, resulting in a 'useless arm'. The arm is not weak in the least, but loss of sense of position and of all the essential information from the muscles and joints makes any co-ordinated movement impossible.

The spinal cord is also involved in the reflexes that control the function of the bladder and bowel and of sexual function in men. These are often disturbed late in the course of the disease, but also occasionally at the onset, even without any other obvious symptoms. This may present with the sudden complete inability to pass urine—acute retention of urine—for some reason virtually always in young women. There are other causes for this uncomfortable event and MS is certainly not the most common. Impotence is a common symptom in the late stage of MS and may rarely be present in the initial attack but I have never encountered this as an isolated symptom of the disease. The importance of this is that men troubled by sexual impotence, who do not have any other symptoms or signs of organic nervous disease do not have MS.

Plaques in the brain stem

The other two common modes of onset are due to plaques in what is known as the brain stem (Plate 7). This is a part of the brain immediately above the spinal cord through which pass all the motor and sensory tracts already mentioned, but which is also crowded with nuclei, or groups of neurones, controlling, among other important functions, the movement of the eyes and the reception of sensory information from the ears.

Double vision

Weakness of one of the six muscles that control the movement of the eyeball causes double vision as the two eyes are no longer always correctly co-ordinated. Double vision as a first symptom of MS is transitory, but always persists for at the very least several days, and therefore does not resemble the momentary double vision of fatigue acting on imperfectly balanced eye muscles that many otherwise normal people experience.

Deafness

For unknown reasons MS plaques only rarely cause deafness, although the brain stem contains nuclei concerned with hearing. The delicate mechanisms of the ear are not, however, solely concerned with hearing but also with balance, and here again the brain stem is an important relay station for nerve impulses serving this function. Giddiness may therefore be the first symptom of MS. I must hasten to qualify this statement, because giddiness of some form or another is an almost universal experience, usually the result of some passing event; an infection, getting out of a hot bath too quickly or having too much to drink, for example. The giddiness of MS is true vertigo, that is to say, an intensely unpleasant and persistent feeling of rotation of the outside world or of oneself often accompanied by vomiting and inability to walk straight, or indeed to walk at all. There are many other causes for vertigo but a young adult prostrated for a week or more, and without other evident cause may well have MS.

Plaques in the cerebellum

Plaques often form in the cerebellum or in the tracts of nerve fibres leading to or from it to other centres in the nervous system; this is more common later in the disease than at the onset. The cerebellum is a complex part of the brain situated at the back of the head, to which information from all the sensory systems is carried, analysed, and used to regulate movement. The effect of interruption of its functions is not to produce loss of any form of sensation, for the cerebellum is not concerned with consciousness, but loss of control of movement. Strength is retained but smooth action of the limbs becomes impossible and movements are said to be un-co-ordinated or ataxic. At the onset of MS this may show itself as unsteadiness in walking or in clumsiness in the use of one or both hands, without weakness or loss of sensation on testing.

Many normal people have shaky hands when agitated or when performing in public, but this can easily be distinguished from the effects of damage to the cerebellum just described.

These then are the common modes of onset of the more usual form of MS, that with remissions and relapses. The list could be extended almost indefinitely with the multitudinous functions of the nervous system, but I am not writing a textbook of neurology. All these modes of onset have features in common. In the first place patients very rarely feel generally unwell. Some authorities have tried to identify even earlier symptoms preceding those clearly indicating organic nervous disease and have written of 'rheumatic' symptoms or headache in particular.

I have not been able to identify anything resembling these joint and muscle pains and have only occasionally encountered headache that I thought might be related to the onset of MS. In the great majority of cases the subject is feeling in perfect health at the time of onset and in particular there is no fever, rash, nor other evidence of a generalized disease. A point of particular interest is that the onset can be extraordinarily rapid. A young woman went to her daughter's school sports and entered for the mother's race feeling very fit and, as she said, intending to win. She ran five yards and then her legs became weak and numb so that she fell down. She was helped up and walked with difficulty, but recovered completely in the course of the next two months. This later proved to have been the initial symptom of MS.

I have described the onset as affecting a single part of the CNS; optic nerve, spinal cord, or brain stem, and this is often so. The disease is, however, *multiple* sclerosis, and even at the onset there may be symptoms and signs of damage to several areas that could not possibly be due to any form of disease confined to a single circumscribed site. Thus a combination of double vision and vertigo with loss of feeling below the waist would clearly indicate disease in both the brain stem and the spinal cord and thus provide evidence of multiple plaques.

In approximately 10 per cent of patients with MS the mode of onset differs from that described above in that it is progressive from the beginning. In many of these patients symptoms begin at a relatively late age, beyond the peak age of those in the early 30s. In this group the first symptom is nearly always gradually progressive weakness of one or both legs. There is nothing resembling an acute attack and unfortunately no remission either. In technical terms these patients have 'progressive spastic paraparesis'.

'Progressive' is self-evident.

'Spastic' refers to the type of weakness that results from interruption of the pyramidal tracts. In addition to weakness of the legs there is loss of control over certain essential automatic reflex actions that are normally carried out through the nervous connections in the spinal cord. These can be tested by the doctor's

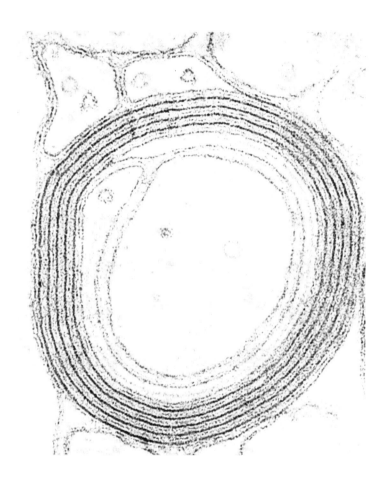

Plate 1. This shows the normal appearance of a nerve fibre or axon surrounded by spiral layers of myelin. This is shown in cross-section enormously magnified under an electron microscope. It is difficult to obtain such beautiful pictures except under experimental conditions and this is a myelinated fibre in a rat. Human fibres are similar but in most there will be many more spiral layers. At the top of the picture is the oligodendrocyte responsible for laying down the myelin sheath.

The picture was published by Dr Hirano in the *Journal of Cell Biology*, 1967, volume 34, p. 555, and is reproduced by permission.

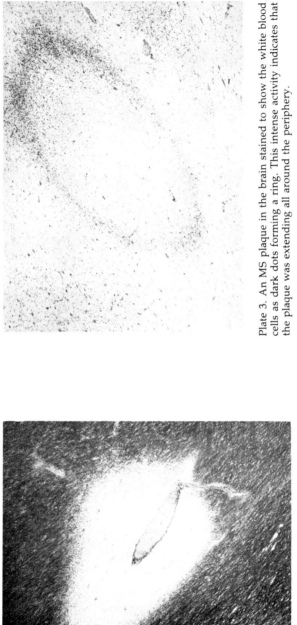

Plate 3. An MS plaque in the brain stained to show the white blood cells as dark dots forming a ring. This intense activity indicates that the plaque was extending all around the periphery.

Plate 2. This is a section of a small plaque. The tissue has been stained so the myelin shows as black, and the sharp contrast between the white plaque and the surrounding normal brain is striking. The magnification is not great enough to show individual nerve fibres. In the centre is a small vein that has been cut across obliquely.

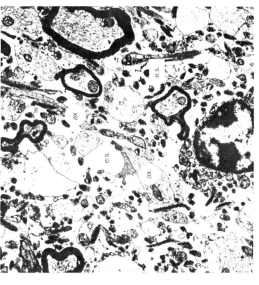

Plate 4(a). This shows an area of the brain in MS tha: has not been involved in a plaque. The black rings are individual myelin sheaths surrounding axons; they are seen in cross-section. The spiral formation cannot be seen in this preparation. The degree of magnification of this electron microscope picture is shown by the bar in the bottom left-hand corner, which indicates how an object one-thousandth of a millimetre in length would appear.
This picture was published by Professor Perier and Dr Gregoir in *Brain*, 1965, volume 88, p. 937 and is reproduced by permission.

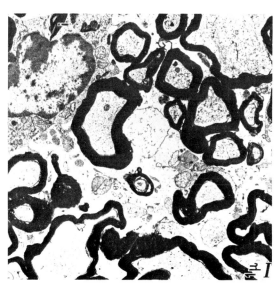

Plate 4(b). This shows, at the same magnification as Plate 4(a), the edge of a plaque. A few battered-looking myelin sheaths can be seen but over most of the area there are bare axons (ax) or spaces (es = extracellular space).
This picture was published by Professor Perier and Dr Gregoir in *Brain*, 1965, volume 88, p. 937 and is reproduced by permission.

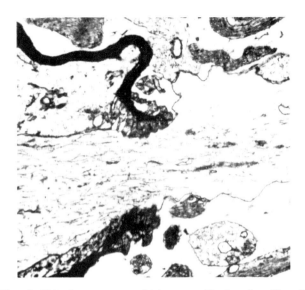

Plate 5. This shows, at even higher magnification than Plate 4(a) and (b), a myelin sheath terminating abruptly in an MS plaque. The axon is seen in longitudinal section running across the picture. The dense black is the myelin sheath, which disappears in the middle of the picture leaving the bare axon bounded by two wavy lines.

This picture was published by Professor Perier and Dr Gregoir in *Brain*, 1965, volume 88, p. 937 and is reproduced by permission.

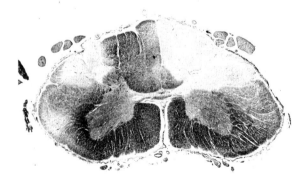

Plate 6. This is a cross-section (about six times life size) of the spinal cord of a patient who had MS. Myelin has been stained black. The large white area in the top right-hand quarter is a plaque that has destroyed myelin in some of the main fibre tracts carrying sensory impulses to the brain. On the other side, two plaques can be seen, one of which, on the extreme left, has involved the main fibre tract carrying impulses concerned with voluntary movement from the brain.

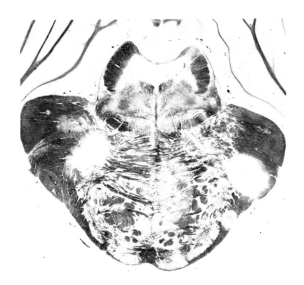

Plate 7(a). This is a cross-section of the brain stem, about twice life size. It is an area packed with nerve fibre tracts passing in both directions between the brain and the spinal cord. The section has been stained so that myelin shows up black. Two punched-out white plaques in which myelin has been destroyed are easily seen.

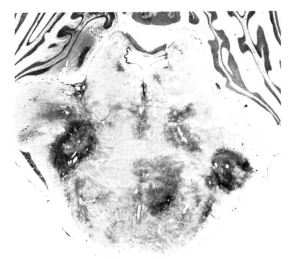

Plate 7(b). The section after Plate 7(a), but now stained so that the scars—the sclerosis—show up black. The two plaques seen in Plate 7(a) are again visible, but there are numerous other scarred areas.

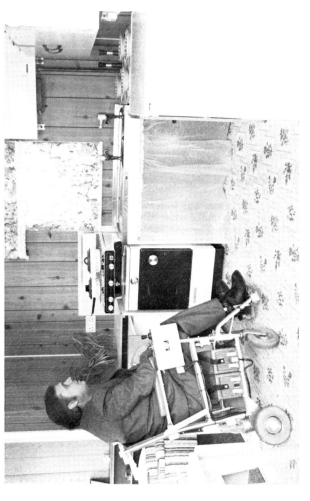

Plate 11. This photograph shows a kitchen that has been adapted for wheelchair use. All the working surfaces are lower than average (about 2 ft 6 in), which means they can be used from a wheelchair with ease and comfort. The cooker is also especially low, enabling someone in a wheelchair to cook safely and independently. Note the low position of the wall cupboards, making them accessible, and the curtain across the bottom of the sink unit, taking the place of cupboards, so that the patient can sit right up to the sink with their knees under the unit. The kitchen shown here has a 4 ft turning circle, allowing a wheelchair to be manoeuvred easily.

rubber hammer of the comic cartoon, which is used to tap the tendons at the knee and ankle to stretch the muscles and induce a reflex contraction. A knee jerk is, as everyone knows, a normal finding, but when the pyramidal tracts are not functioning normally in MS or in other diseases the knee jerk is much increased. In itself this is of little consequence, but is an indication of abnormally increased reflex activity, so that stretching the muscles in ordinary movement also causes exaggerated reflex contraction. Sometimes a repetitive reflex may be set up, particularly in the calf muscles, resulting in an effect perhaps best described as 'juddering'. This may first show itself when the foot is firmly pressed on the brake pedal of a car. The calf muscles are stretched and contract reflexly, causing a jerk, and this is repeated for as long as pressure is maintained. The technical name for this is *clonus*. The result of these increased reflexes is a stiff 'spastic' leg and the patient scrapes the toe on walking and drags the limb. The abnormality also shows itself in an abnormal reaction to firm stroking of the sole of the foot when the toes normally reflexly curl under, but in a spastic leg they stretch out in the opposite direction. Many people find this test unpleasant but it is of considerable value in diagnosis. It is virtually impossible to elicit this reflex on oneself and self-examination is to be deprecated.

The word 'paraparesis' means weakness of both legs and is a milder form of the more familiar paraplegia used when there is complete paralysis such as may follow injury to the spinal cord.

The symptoms and signs as described above are present alone or in combination at the onset of the disease in perhaps 85 per cent of cases, the remainder having other symptoms more commonly encountered later in the course of the disease, which I will describe in Chapter 4.

4 *The course of the disease*

One of the most remarkable facts about MS is the astonishing variability in its course and severity. Some variation is of course not unusual in chronic disease. Rheumatoid arthritis, for example, may be either mild or severe throughout its course or show great fluctuations, including complete remission. Some chronic infections such as tuberculosis can remain dormant for many years before eventually causing overt disease. Parallels can therefore be drawn from other diseases, but none approaches the vagaries of the natural history of MS that never cease to surprise the neurologist even after a lifetime of experience. The course of MS varies from that of an obviously grave disease to a literally imperceptible condition discovered accidentally after death from unrelated causes in old age. Between these two extremes lie the great majority of cases, but even here there is great variation in the speed of progression and eventual outcome.

The existence of a benign form is little known and certainly requires emphasis but if MS were no more than a mild nuisance there would be little point in writing a book about it. It would be futile to attempt to conceal the well-known fact that MS is often a crippling disease, causing severe disability in previously healthy young adults. It has been urged on me that to describe the clinical details of MS for non-medical readers will inexcusably cause depression and distress, but I think this unlikely. With few exceptions I have found that people with MS have a strong and justified desire to know the truth and are ready to face the facts bravely. I shall therefore begin by describing the typical course of a moderately severe case.

Initial stage

The person, most often a woman around the age of 30, has an initial attack as described in Chapter 2, optic neuritis, numbness, weakness, double vision, or any of a great number of other less frequently encountered symptoms, either separately or in different combinations. Recovery is complete within a few weeks and all is apparently well. A diagnosis may not have been made or even suspected and the disease has now become latent.

Relapses

After an interval of from several months to several years new symptoms develop, usually different from those of the initial attack. Thus optic neuritis may be followed by numbness or weakness of the legs and again recovery is complete. A further relapse, this time more severe and often including weakness of both legs, occurs within the succeeding year or two and this time recovery is not complete—there are permanent symptoms and permanent slight disability, amounting perhaps to weakness of one leg when tired and inability to run. This pattern of successive relapses once or twice a year or once in two years may persist for a further three or four years, each time with less complete recovery and increasing residual symptoms. Eventually a stage is reached in which there is persistent difficulty in walking due to a combination of the spastic weakness and ataxia described in Chapter 3. The hands may also be a little tremulous and unsteady. Eyesight is usually normal but there will by now almost certainly be symptoms of that most distressing disability, failure of the normal control of the urinary bladder. A normal adult can, within wide limits, decide when and when not to pass urine. Control is exercised by the brain through connections in the spinal cord and it is these that are damaged in MS. A usual result is that *reflex* emptying of the bladder takes over, that is to say, when filling reaches a certain pressure the bladder automatically empties. In the early stages voluntary control is not entirely lost. The reflex activity is heightened so that the desire to pass urine becomes urgent when there is only a small quantity in the bladder. This urgency may lead to incontinence if there is no convenient lavatory. Less often it becomes difficult to start to pass urine in spite of a strong desire to do so or the two conditions, urgency and hesitancy, may alternate.

At this stage sexual potency in the male often declines. There is no reduction in desire but ability to sustain an erection fails and intercourse becomes infrequent and unsatisfactory.

MS is often accompanied by a degree of fatigue seemingly quite out of proportion to any physical disability that may be present. Indeed, undue fatigue may occur as an early symptom when the diagnosis is still in doubt. Tiredness is, however, a sensation familiar to many people not suffering from any disease at all and, in the absence of other relevant symptoms, should not give rise to any suspicion of MS.

A matter of obvious practical importance is the recognition of immediate precipitating causes of relapse. Many have been proposed, among them emotional disturbance, acute infections, injuries, exposure to cold, excessive exertion and fatigue, surgical operations, and pregnancy. Every neurologist will have records of striking individual examples in which one of these factors has immediately preceded a relapse, but no general pattern emerges. There are unavoidable fallacies in trying to investigate these possibilities in retrospect, for there is a natural tendency to remember or to exaggerate events that have an apparent relationship in time to the onset of an illness and to forget the rest. For the great majority of relapses no precipitating cause can be found.

Some less common symptoms

I must describe some less common or less obtrusive symptoms that may be of great importance to individual patients. MS is not an intrinsically painful disease but in certain circumstances pain may be experienced. Backache is common and is due to the strain and excessive use put on the back muscles by walking with weak and spastic legs. It is seldom severe or persistent. If spasticity is severe in later stages of the disease there may be sudden spasms in which the legs either shoot out straight or bend sharply at the knee and hip, particularly in bed at night. Usually these are no more than annoying but the latter form, flexor spasms, are sometimes painful. Neither the spasm nor the backache are specific for MS but may occur in any condition causing spastic weakness of the legs.

There is a rare form of persistent pain, usually in one arm or in some area of the trunk or in both feet, that does appear to be directly due to some effect of MS on the nervous system, but little is known of how it is caused. More common and more important is the condition known as trigeminal neuralgia, often referred to by the French descriptive title of *tic douloureux*, invariably mispronounced as something like 'dolorou'. The nerve that carries sensory impulses from the face is called the trigeminal nerve because it has three branches. Neuralgia is an old-fashioned but useful word meaning 'nerve pain'. The French name includes the pain and also the '*tic*' or involuntary contraction of the face during the attack of pain. Trigeminal neuralgia usually has nothing to do with MS and occurs, for no discoverable reason, in middle-aged or elderly people who have no other evidence of nervous disease. When it occurs in young people it may be the first symptom of MS or it may develop at any stage of the disease.

The pain is quite characteristic, being felt in a restricted area of one side of the face, in sudden brief paroxysms of great severity. Many of these are brought on, or triggered, by touching the face as in washing, shaving or applying make up, or by eating or talking. Each attack lasts no more than 10 or 15 seconds but is often agonizing and is accompanied by the '*tic*' or grimace. It occurs many times a day. Apart from the fact that, as described in Chapter 8, it can be most sucessfully treated, the interest of trigeminal neuralgia in MS is that it seems to be quite a different *kind* of symptom from the familiar weakness and numbness due to failure of demyelinated axons to conduct the nervous impulse. Indeed there seems to be *excessive* conduction, many axons firing off abnormally and simultaneously.

There are a number of similar paroxysmal symptoms in MS, although they are less well known than trigeminal neuralgia because they are in general much less painful. They include brief episodes of unsteadiness, slurred speech or cramp-like contractions of the hand or foot. A symptom recently recognized is paroxysms of intense itching confined to some isolated area of skin. They all have the same characteristics of being triggered by movement, lasting no more than a minute or two and occurring with great frequency for a few weeks before going into remission. They can also be instantly prevented by the same treatment that controls trigeminal neuralgia. It is likely that all result from a similar effect of demyelination. The nerve impulse carried along an axon is normally effectively isolated or insulated from neighbouring axons and, indeed, it is difficult to imagine that the nervous system could function if this was not so. Loss of the myelin sheath from axons still capable of conducting could lead to the nerve impulse spreading sideways to other axons, causing a sudden massive discharge and the paroxysm of pain, itching, or muscle contraction.

A curious symptom often present at some stage of MS consists of a surge of pins and needles down the back and legs on bending the neck. In the days when men wore short hair this was sometimes called the 'barber's chair sign' as it would be experienced when the head was bent forward for the application of clippers. It is seldom more than a mild nuisance.

The effect of temperature

Many people with MS become aware of a pronounced effect of temperature on their symptoms. A hot day, a hot bath, exertion, or even a hot drink may cause temporary weakness or blurring of vision. Some people find this so unpleasant that they never have the bath water more than tepid and learn to dread heat waves. The effect does not last for long; a woman told me that after a hot bath she would be unable to read in bed for about three-quarters of an hour. The beneficial effect of cold is less obvious, partly because this may actually aggravate spasticity so that any improvement in strength would be masked and such patients actually prefer hot weather. These effects of heat are readily explicable as there is experimental evidence that even a minute rise in temperature will increase the proportion of demyelinated axons that cannot conduct at all. The effect is not harmful and these brief reversible increases in symptoms are quite different from an acute relapse.

The effect of MS on the mind

A natural concern of anyone with MS is whether it will affect the mind. As will be described, it is undeniable that in the terminal stages of the severe form of the disease there is some impairment of memory and of the power of reasoning, and indeed rigorous testing may show minor changes at an earlier stage. The great majority of those with MS are mentally normal throughout virtually the whole course of the disease. It is only natural that some should be depressed but this is not obviously more common than in the rest of the population and most remain calm and philosophical about their disabilities and prospects. This admirable stoicism is distinct from the abnormal cheerfulness or euphoria sometimes seen in those with blunted mental acuity.

Other symptoms of MS

Other symptoms can be mentioned more briefly. MS does not cause permanent deafness and only rarely has even any temporary effect on the hearing. Severe and permanent damage to the vision in both eyes is fortunately rare. Epileptic fits hardly ever result from MS and persistent recurrent epilepsy probably does not occur.

Later stages of MS

After the active stage of relapse and remission lasting for about five years the pattern often changes and there are no more acute attacks and no more spontaneous recovery. Symptoms and actual capacity for such exertions as climbing stairs often fluctuate a great deal from day to day and in the course of the day, being influenced by fatigue, temperature, and other unknown factors. These variations are quite different in timing and in significance to the acute relapse lasting for several weeks. Many people now experience a long period extending over many years during which their symptoms and degree of disability do not change significantly beyond these expected fluctuations. They can walk, although not easily, can drive a suitable vehicle, and can work or cope with the household and children with no more than family support. Life is a struggle but by no means intolerable.

Eventually if the disease is indeed in the severe form this static period will be followed by a progressive stage. Walking becomes increasingly difficult. Sticks are no longer adequate support and recourse must be had to a walking frame or to holding on to furniture. A wheelchair becomes necessary for outdoor excursions and eventually at home as well. Bladder control is increasingly lost with resulting incontinence but some degree of bowel control is usually retained, although constipation may be uncomfortable. The hands and arms become increasingly shaky and ataxic in such activities as holding a cup or a spoon. This may become a severe disability quite out of proportion to any weakness of the limbs. It is referred to as 'intention tremor' because it becomes evident or increases whenever some voluntary action is attempted. Eyesight may deteriorate, either because of further damage to the optic nerves or because the eyes oscillate instead of remaining fixed on the object of regard. This is called nystagmus and in MS is due to damage to the cerebellum or the tracts connecting it to the brain stem, producing a sort of ataxia of movements of the eyes.

I have hesitated to describe the final stages of the severe form of MS, but the purpose of this book is to convey the facts of what is already universally known to be potentially a grave disease. Increasing damage to spinal cord and brain leads to a bedridden and helpless state and, at this stage, mental powers are undoubtedly affected. Memory and concentration fail and it is now that the so-called euphoria may be seen. This literally means a sense of well-being, which must indeed be rare but it is common to see patients cheerful and apparently indifferent to severe disabilities. With careful nursing, either in hospital, disabled unit, or at home, the risks inherent in the bedridden and incontinent state can be held at bay for many years but eventually infection spreads from the paralysed bladder to the kidneys, pneumonia assails the lungs, or intractable bedsores develop and in turn become infected. It is these complications that are the immediate cause of death.

At the other extreme of recognizable MS is the benign form. The symptoms at the onset are entirely typical of MS but are often confined to attacks of retrobulbar neuritis and of numbness and tingling of the limbs and trunk. Remission is complete, even after many relapses, and severe disability or indeed any form of permanent disability at all does not develop. I have known people who have come to regard it as quite normal that they should have one or two episodes of loss of sensation of some part of the limbs or trunk two or three times a year. Others may have no more than two relapses or perhaps even a single attack, typical of the disease, but entirely without recurrence. Others again may have infrequent relapses at intervals of many years. In one of my patients 25 symptomfree years elapsed between two typical attacks of MS. In a rather less benign form some permanent symptoms, such as dragging of one leg, are present after a few years but are insufficient to interfere with work or with the enjoyment of life.

The outcome of MS

Everyone with MS will rightly want to know the eventual outcome, but it is seldom possible to be in any way precise in the early years of the disease. Certainly there are definite indications of a relatively bad result. When MS is progressive from the onset without remission and relapse it usually takes the severe form. As these people are often older than the average age for the onset of the disease it follows that, in general, the older the age of onset, the worse the outlook, but of course there are exceptions. Another indication of a poor outlook is an initial severe attack with incomplete recovery. The indications of a benign course are less distinctive. Symptoms confined to those of damage to the optic nerve or the sensory pathways of the spinal cord, with little or no weakness or ataxia are, in general, favourable signs, but unfortunately only in a statistical sense, rather than providing a definite forecast in individuals. Figures are indeed available but these are of little use or interest to someone who has just recovered from a second relapse and wants to plan for the future. These figures are also necessarily an approximation. As explained in the next chapter, diagnosis of the mild or early case or of progressive disease is often difficult and figures are bound to be weighted by severe cases where the diagnosis has been established for many years.

Anyone describing the outcome in MS is bound to acknowledge a debt to those who have had the energy and interest to follow and record the progress of their patients over 25 years or more. The conclusions are in broad agreement. The average duration of life after the onset of symptoms is at least 25 years. In 5 per cent or less of cases the disease takes on a particularly severe form in which death may result within 5 years from involvement of centres in the brain stem controlling breathing and other vital functions but this form is distinctly rare. The proportion of those with the benign form shows some decline with increasing duration of the disease, showing that the benign course may after many years eventually become progressive. According to one estimate, 10 years after the first symptom one-third of all those known to have MS will have little or no disability, reducing to one-quarter after 15 years and to one in five after 20 years. These figures are almost certainly unduly pessimistic, as another investigator found that 50 per cent of men with MS lived for more than 35 years after the onset. If disability remains slight 5 years after the first symptom other than optic neuritis the disease often remains mild but, as usual, there are exceptions.

5 *The diagnosis of multiple sclerosis*

It might well be thought that any doctor familiar with the facts outlined in preceding chapters would have no difficulty in correctly diagnosing MS, but this is far from being so. In some instances the diagnosis is, indeed, obvious enough, but even here some caution is advisable. In series of published case histories the average interval between the first symptom and diagnosis being made is several years. Early symptoms, such as pins and needles, even if unduly persistent, are often ignored or, if the doctor is consulted, are misinterpreted. It must be remembered that no general practitioner has much opportunity to obtain extensive personal experience of the more difficult aspects of the disease. When confronted by someone complaining of tingling or numbness of strange distribution in whom no weakness or change in the reflexes conventionally examined can be found, it is not too difficult to believe that the patient, usually a young woman, is being 'hysterical'. The numbness complained of may be hard to detect by the usual methods of testing with pin pricks and cotton wool. An experienced neurologist will recognize that when told that the pin feels sharp, but that in some way as if there is something between the pin and the skin, this is a genuine disturbance of sensation, but it undoubtedly sounds peculiar and can lead to misunderstanding. Even if MS is considered possible there is a natural reluctance to make the diagnosis, as nobody likes to be the bearer of bad news. Apart from some special circumstances, there is at present no great virtue in establishing an *early* diagnosis but when effective treatment is discovered it will certainly be best applied early in the course of the disease before irreparable loss of axons has occurred.

The diagnosis of MS is usually made on clinical grounds, that is to say, by finding the symptoms and signs of damage to more than one area of the central nervous system, occurring at more than one time. There are, however, a number of other diseases that do exactly this and that must be distinguished from MS. This may be difficult in the first attack and also in the 10 per cent of instances of MS where the symptoms point to progressive damage at a single site, often the spinal cord. There is an obvious need for ways of confirming the diagnosis made on the clinical features. Despite claims to the contrary there is no test that is 100 per cent reliable in showing whether MS is or is not present. This should not cause surprise, as it is the case for many diseases. In MS there have been great advances towards such certainty and these are described later in this chapter, but first it is important to consider a few of the conditions that may be mistaken for MS. A complete list of these would be absurdly long and technical and I will not attempt it.

Diseases that mimic MS

Diseases that can occasionally closely mimic the relapsing and remitting form of MS belong to the small print sections reserved for rarities in large medical textbooks, rather than in a book intended for general reading, but it is interesting to consider how any possible diagnostic confusion could arise. These conditions, which can be simply listed for the curious as sarcoidosis, systemic lupus erythematosus and chronic Lyme disease, produce most of their adverse effects on the nervous system by interfering with its blood supply. Small arteries become blocked because of inflammation and thickening of their walls, and scattered areas of the central nervous system are damaged because of lack of oxygen normally carried by the blood.

An early theory had attributed the scattered plaques of MS to the blocking of small blood vessels, in this case veins. Although this could never be substantiated and appears to have been incorrect, it was at least a plausible way in which multiple damage to the central nervous system might have been caused. A stroke, due to blocking of an artery by a blood clot, is uncommon at the usual age of onset of MS, but may cause symptoms almost indistinguishable from those of a first attack of MS. Surprisingly, confusion has sometimes resulted from common symptoms of the distressing but essentially harmless condition of classic migraine. In many sufferers the headache is preceded by numbness and tingling in one arm, but this lasts for no more than 20 minutes and should not give rise to any problem in diagnosis.

However, in most cases of MS the diagnosis is not in serious doubt for long. Far more difficult are the problems posed by the progressive form of the disease. Here there is no doubt at all that there is progressive disease of the nervous system, most frequently involving mainly or exclusively the spinal cord. The problem is to avoid overlooking some quite different disease requiring entirely different management. The most common source of error is to confuse MS of this type with the effects of compression of the spinal cord by a tumour or prolapsed intervertebral disc. MS may be suspected but it is so important not to overlook a tumour of this kind that can be removed with resulting complete cure that thorough investigation is often necessary to ensure that no such mistake has been made. As an example, many years ago I was asked to see a young woman diagnosed as having MS who had been advised not to have any children. She was pregnant and was naturally anxious and concerned. I was able to show that she had a benign cause of spinal cord compression, which was removed successfully, resulting in a cure of her symptoms and also allowing her to complete the pregnancy and have her much-wanted baby. Such happy results are uncommon and, in most patients investigated, no cause of spinal cord compression is found.

Other forms of chronic nervous disease that may be confused with the progressive type of MS include a group of hereditary diseases that result in a variety of symptoms and signs due to degeneration in the spinal cord and cerebellum. On the whole the outcome in these diseases is less favourable than in MS but it is important to establish the correct diagnosis because advice will be needed about the risks of transmitting hereditary disease to succeeding generations. Inborn, congenital abnormalities of the cerebellum and upper part of the spinal cord can some-times produce symptoms for the first time in adult life and these, again, must not be overlooked, as surgical treatment may be helpful. The accurate recognition of another form of spinal cord degeneration is even more important. This is the spinal cord damage that can result from deficiency of vitamin B_{12}. For practical purposes this results from failure to absorb the vitamin and not from a deficient diet. The usual result is pernicious anaemia, but in some patients the spinal cord damage pre-dominates, with symptoms of tingling and weakness in the legs. Patients are usually older than those with MS but the symptoms could otherwise easily cause confusion. Deficiency of vitamin B_{12} can be diagnosed by finding a low level of the vitamin in the blood. If treated in time by injections of the missing vitamin recovery is complete and to misdiagnose this condition as MS is a serious error. A full discussion of the differential diagnosis of MS would obviously be inappropriate and the investigation of the progressive or unusual case can be complex and incon-clusive. Enough has been said to illustrate the need for some more positive method of diagnosis than simply the history of the disease and the findings on examination.

A test for MS?

There is no specific test for MS. This is not surprising, as the same is also true of many diseases affecting many different systems of the body. The positive diagnosis of many diseases depends on identifying the nature of infecting bacteria or viruses or on examining a portion of the affected tissue under the microscope. MS, whatever else it is, is certainly no ordinary infection and it is not practicable nor sensible to remove parts of the brain on the chance of finding an MS plaque. Even when the symptoms and signs are strongly suggestive of MS it is usual and sensible to seek confirmation or otherwise of the diagnosis from laboratory tests. Considerable advances have been made in this direction.

The central nervous system is surrounded by a clear watery fluid known as the cerebrospinal fluid. This can easily be examined without risk by means of a procedure known as lumbar puncture. This is traditionally regarded by patients with dread, reflected perhaps in the common misnomer 'lumbar punch', but when skilfully performed with a very fine needle it is almost or completely painless. The membranes enclosing the fluid extend further down the spine than does the spinal cord and the needle can be inserted between two of the lumbar vertebrae in the low back, and the specimen of fluid withdrawn. An occasional undesirable effect is an unpleasant headache for a day or two. It used to be claimed that lumbar puncture precipitated relapse in MS but I do not believe this to be true. In MS there is often a slight increase in the small number of white blood cells (lymphocytes) present in the fluid and also an increase in the level of protein, which is normally very low in comparison to the blood. These changes are inconstant and are certainly not diagnostic of MS but the investigation is still useful, as in some other diseases that might be confused with MS the changes are much more marked.

More important is the nature of the protein in the fluid. This can be examined by electrophoresis, which is a method of displaying the different types of protein present according to their molecular weight. In about 90 per cent of people with MS the globulin protein in the fluid can be shown by this method to contain one or several concentrations not normally present. These show up as bands on the blotting paper used in the test and are known as oligoclonal bands. These bands are not, unfortunately, specific for MS but, in the context of appropriate symptoms, go some way towards confirming the diagnosis, while their absence may cause some doubts.

Quite different techniques, made possible by developments in electronics, are now used extensively. It is now possible to record from the surface of the scalp or the skin of the neck the minute electrical potentials induced or evoked by stimulation of some form of sensory inflow to the central nervous system. The response to a single stimulus cannot be detected as it is swamped by background 'noise' arising from contraction of muscles, spontaneous electrical activity in the nervous system, and other unwanted interference. If, however, the responses to several hundred stimuli are averaged they can be seen clearly while all random activity is cancelled out. This involves the recording apparatus being triggered by the stimulus so that the expected response always appears at the same point on the sweep of the recording oscilloscope. The normal response to stimulating the retina can be recorded over the back of the head near the centres in the brain concerned with vision and is shown in Plate 8. The most constant wave in normal subjects is the downward deflection that occurs about 100 milliseconds (i.e. $1/10$ of a second) after the stimulus. In this illustration the responses to 250 stimuli resulting from a chequerboard pattern alternating once a second have been averaged. The nervous pathways between the retina and the visual centres in the occipital lobes at the back of the brain are long and complex but of course include the optic nerves so frequently involved in plaques of MS.

The first step was to show that during an attack of optic neuritis the main electrical potential evoked at 100 milliseconds was of low voltage and abnormally long latency, that is to say it did not occur at 100 milliseconds from the stimulus but at perhaps 150 milliseconds or even later. This was interesting but not altogether surprising as an expected result of demyelination would be the slowing of nervous conduction in just this way. What was surprising was that this delay in conduction persisted in most cases after the vision in the affected eye had recovered and, indeed, indefinitely. Here then, was a method of detecting the effects of demyelination in the *absence of relevant symptoms*. It had long been suspected that plaques occurred in the optic nerve without producing a recognizable attack of neuritis and, indeed, without any complaint from the patient at all. In patients with MS the head of the optic nerve as seen through an ophthalmoscope often looks abnormally pale, whether or not there is a history of optic neuritis in the past and despite quite normal eyesight. The next step was to use this evoked potential technique in people with symptoms of progressive disease of the spinal cord in an attempt to show *multiple* lesions, that is to say unsuspected symptomless areas of damage in the optic nerves, in addition to the obvious one in the spinal cord. Considerable success has been achieved by this method but, again, a positive result has not been obtained in more than two-thirds of patients with MS.

Other forms of nerve stimulation and appropriate recording have also been used. An astonishing series of minute electrical potentials can be averaged following stimulation of the ear by a repetitive click. Electrical stimulation of a nerve in the arm evokes a recognizable response in the neck and over the scalp related to conduction in the sensory nervous pathways through the spinal cord to the brain. Both these forms of evoked potential can be disturbed in MS, even when the patient has no symptoms that would in any way lead one to suspect that such abnormalities were present.

In a few hospitals a method involving stimulating through the intact scalp and skull the area of the brain concerned with movement of the limbs by means of a magnetic field. The timing of the response in the muscles can be measured and this may be delayed in MS. How often this can show up abnormalities that could not be found by ordinary medical examination is not entirely clear.

By far the most important advance has been the discovery of means of 'imaging' the substance of the brain and, to a lesser extent, of the spinal cord. Computerized tomography (CT scanning) is a method of analysing multiple X-ray exposures so as to build up pictures of the brain as seen in slices (Plate 9). This technique revolutionized the ease of diagnosis of many diseases of the central nervous system and spared many patients from undergoing much more unpleasant X-ray investigations. It was capable of showing on X-ray film areas of abnormality in the brain in MS, particularly when the scan was 'enhanced' by the injection into a vein of iodine-containing substances that accumulated in the damaged areas and were opaque to X-rays. However, positive results were only found in about 40 per cent of people known to have MS and where the diagnosis was doubtful the proportion was much lower.

This method of imaging was soon superseded by magnetic resonance imaging (MRI). This technique does not involve X-rays but uses a powerful magnetic field. This causes all the hydrogen atoms in the organ being examined—the brain or spinal cord—to orientate themselves in line with the field. A brief burst of radio-frequency waves is then passed through, disturbing this orientation. When the burst is switched off the spinning hydrogen atoms re-adjust to the magnetic field, sending off radio waves that can be recorded on film. As most of the hydrogen atoms in the brain are found in water molecules, an increased signal on MRI means that the water content of the area giving off the signal must be abnormally high and, in MS, what is seen on the film is either swelling in an acute plaque or fluid replacing the normal tissues that have been lost in chronic plaques. The technique can be adjusted in many ways according to what it is hoped to show on the films. Few non-specialists, including myself, find the physics of MRI easy to understand. The apparatus is very expensive to buy and to maintain but MRI has contributed greatly to the understanding of MS and to ease of diagnosis. It is painless although some people feel unpleasantly boxed in, and the scan is rather noisy. It has the added advantage of having no known adverse side-effects.

MRI is far more sensitive than CT scanning and in people with established MS shows up a great many more unsuspected abnormalities in the brain (Plate 10). With recent developments it is even possible to show abnormalities in the optic nerves and in the spinal cord. Even in very early disease, when the first symptoms may be those of a single area of damage to the nervous system, such as optic neuritis, multiple abnormalities can often be seen, not giving rise to any symptoms, thus establishing that disease is present at *multiple* sites when this could not have been suspected from the symptoms alone. There is, however, a snag; these changes are seen not only in MS but also, less frequently, and usually less typically, in a number of other diseases that might be mistaken for MS.

Unfortunately not one of these tests is genuinely specific for MS and it would also be perfectly possible to have MS and to show no abnormality at all in any of these investigations. This is not surprising or out of keeping with what is found in many important diseases: there is no infallible test for coronary thrombosis or cancer, for example.

Increased certainty of diagnosis is greatly to be desired, not only because people have a right to know what is wrong with them and doctors like to know what they are trying to treat, but because understanding of the disease must depend on accurate information.

6 The cause of multiple sclerosis

Despite many years of intense and accelerating research the cause of MS remains unknown. Before considering the many theories that have been advanced and those currently under investigation it is important to consider briefly what is really meant by 'cause' in medicine. Often enough there seems to be no problem—the influenza virus causes an attack of influenza, although why you, rather than your neighbour, should catch it may not be so simple. In many diseases, however, causation must be regarded as a chain that may be followed link by link, but seldom for very far. For example, a coronary thrombosis or a stroke is usually due to hardening of the arteries or high blood pressure, but the causes of these, where known at all, are what it is now fashionable to call multifactorial. Risk factors that increase the chance of having arteriosclerosis or of suffering from its effects can be identified—bad heredity, advancing age, perhaps an injudicious diet, obesity, and cigarette smoking—but a single underlying reason why cholesterol is laid down in the walls of the arteries has not been found and perhaps does not exist. We should not therefore be too surprised or disheartened by the present failure to identify a cause of MS. What is needed is to follow the chain of causation back to a point at which effective treatment or prevention can be applied. There are many examples in medicine where this has been done, perhaps most remarkably in diabetes. The reason why insulin is not secreted normally in this disease is not fully known, but this has not prevented the development of treatment that has entirely transformed the life of diabetic patient. Smallpox vaccination was effective long before viruses were ever heard of. Successful treatment or prevention of MS need not depend on fully unravelling the cause but perhaps on the discovery of but one further link in the chain.

The quest for the cause or causes of MS has certainly not failed for lack of volume of information, such a mass of data has accumulated that it is possible to select facts to fit virtually any theory propounded. There are, however, certain facts that surely must be explained in any finally convincing solution. These include the strange geographical distribution, the age range, the increased incidence in families, and the pattern of relapse and remission. Individually these can all be matched by other diseases but taken together they form a unique pattern. The need to explain these facts is of course known to all serious investigators who have indeed often used them as the starting point of their working theories.

However distasteful the idea of animal experimentation, it is unfortunately true that many advances in medicine would not have progressed very far without the use of laboratory animals. MS is, however, exclusively a human disease and there is no natural equivalent in animals. This has a limiting effect on research, as observation in animals of the factors that cause relapse and the effect of treatment would almost certainly be illuminating.

There is, however, another approach. It has long been known that there is another demyelinating disease of man, much less common than MS and differing in several ways. This is called *acute disseminated encephalomyelitis*, which simply means that there are scattered areas of inflammation in the brain and spinal cord; inflammation surrounding small veins and accompanied by demyelination, recognizably similar to the lesions of MS. This disease, however, nearly always follows some definite infection such as measles, chickenpox, or smallpox vaccination. With very few exceptions it does not relapse. The patient either recovers completely, dies in the acute stage, or recovers with some residual evidence of damage to the central nervous system, but in any event there is no recurrence. There is no reasonable doubt that this demyelinating disease has been produced in experimental animals but not by ordinary infection.

Allergy and autoimmunity

One possible mechanism of production of the lesions of MS that has long been under investigation is that of allergy. This is a difficult concept to explain and, as applied to MS, has little resemblance to such well-known afflictions as sensitivity to pollen resulting in hay fever. The demyelinating disease in animals that resembles acute disseminated encephalomyelitis has been produced by the injection of extracts of tissues of the central nervous system itself, combined with other agents that enhance the effect. The result appears to be to render the animal's nervous system allergic to some component of the central nervous system and, as the animal naturally has its own central nervous system, the allergy extends to its own tissues. This phenomenon is known as *autoimmunity* and means that the immune mechanisms that normally act to reject foreign invaders such as germs react in the same way to some normal constituent of the body and destroy it. These mechanisms are complex. Certain cells in the body can manufacture antibodies—chemicals that circulate in the blood and react specifically with and neutralize the foreign material that stimulated their production. Other protective activities depend on the more direct actions of lymphocytes. In experimental allergic encephalomyelitis (EAE) induced in animals it is the myelin that is destroyed and the animal's nervous system has become allergic to some chemical component of its own myelin, probably to the protein it contains.

Controversy has long raged as to how relevant this EAE is to human MS. A stumbling block has been that, like the human encephalomyelitis that occurs after infection, the animal disease seemed to be self-limiting. By changes in technique, however, it is now possible to produce in small animals a *spontaneously relapsing and remitting disease* without any further injections of brain tissue. This obviously suggests that at last we may have a disease in animals that could be of enormous value in research. For example, methods of treatment could be tried out at no risk to patients and with an answer obtained much more rapidly. The idea that the breakdown of myelin in MS is due to autoimmunity, that is to say, the rejection by the body of its own myelin, has many attractions. The lymphocytes that are so prominent in an acute MS plaque are known to be involved in immune reactions and perhaps this could also be a link with the raised level of immunoglobulins in the cerebrospinal fluid mentioned in Chapter 5. There is, however, one important distinction between MS, the post-infective encephalomyelitis in man, and the allergic disease of animals, in that no cause for the induction of autoimmunity is evident; the patient with MS has not been injected with myelin protein. Even if it is accepted that the immediate cause of the MS plaque is an autoimmune reaction, the chain of causation has not been traced far enough, and the question obviously arises as to why this occurs. It is now generally accepted that there are two essential factors, environmental and genetic; in other words, some external agent acting on an inborn susceptibility.

Environmental factors

The importance of the environmental factor has recently been shown by study of the effects of migration. MS is almost certainly a rare disease in the West Indies and remains so in those who migrate to Britain as adults. In their children, born in Britain and now reaching the usual age of onset of MS, the disease is as common as in the general population. Results of other migrations strongly suggest that whatever the hostile factor in the environment may be, it acts in childhood, many years before any symptoms develop.

The most reliable figures are from Israel and from Hawaii, both areas of relatively low risk with good medical services and doctors familiar with MS. In both there has been an influx of migrants from areas of high MS risk—northern Europe and the United States of America. The results show that those who move in adult life take their high risk with them, while those who migrate in childhood acquire the low risk of their new home. The cut-off point was at first thought to be around the age of 15 but up-to-date results suggest that it may be much younger and perhaps only those who migrate below the age of 5 escape the high risk of their native land. Whichever figure is correct the implication is plain; something happens in early life that determines the chance of acquiring MS. This event, whatever it is, does not occur at birth or apparently in the first few years of childhood because it can be largely avoided by leaving the high risk area within those years. Afterwards it is too late; the event, which seems to depend on environment in high risk countries, has already taken place.

The external factor remains unknown but there is no lack of candidates. More rational suggestions are of excess, deficiency, imbalance in the diet, or infection.

The effect of diet

As an example of the former there have been repeated attempts to incriminate the role of what are known as trace metals in the diet (elements such as copper or zinc that are essential to life but only in minute quantities), or lead, which is undeniably toxic, not least to the nervous system. None of these theories has been supported by detailed investigation, but this does not mean that the influence of these metals can be entirely discarded as this is a difficult field of experimentation. Out of a large number of scientific papers of variable worth one alone seems to have remained as a kind of folk memory in the medical profession. This concerns a curious observation on a disease of myelin in lambs called, in the usual expressive veterinary way, 'swayback'. This was plainly shown to be due to deficiency of copper in the diet of the pregnant ewes, a finding of some importance in animal husbandry. A number of those working on this project developed MS, although how analysing the soil of the sheep pasture could lead to copper deficiency or any other means of transmitting a demyelinating disease was not explained or even reasonably conjectured.

An external poison?	The possibility of an external poison is not to be lightly dismissed. There are many examples of damage to the nervous system, either peripheral or central, arising in this way. Mercury poisoning from industrial pollution has caused a serious disease of the central nervous system in Japan, but there is no evidence that the mercury in dental fillings causes MS, as some have feared. More extensive, but almost confined to Japan, was an epidemic of a disease now known simply as

SMON from the initials of its complex (English) name, subacute myelo-optico-neuropathy. This disease, which in some respects resembles MS, is probably due to excessive consumption of the drug clioquinol, sold under the name of Enterovioform. The Japanese certainly used this drug to a far greater extent than other people, apparently because of a somewhat obsessive attitude to their bowels, but there is more than a hint that they were in some way unduly susceptible to its effects. Many attempts have naturally been made to detect some poisonous agent in the diet or drinking water as the cause for MS, encouraged by the extraordinary geographical distribution. Lead poisoning was once a serious suspect but now seems improbable.

Animal fat   A more serious contender that will be discussed in Chapter 7 is the consumption of animal fat. Enthusiasts have maintained for many years that a high consumption of dairy fat is related to a high incidence of MS but most of this evidence is unconvincing. The original observation was that in Norway the incidence of MS was lower in some fishing communities where little dairy fat is eaten, compared with agricultural villages inland where consumption is high. Whatever its role, dietary animal fat cannot be the sole factor, as MS is rare in some communities where consumption is high, as in the white population of South Africa.

Infection

There is increasing evidence that the external environmental factor involved is some form of infection. Not unnaturally, any mention of infection leads people to think of familiar infectious diseases, diseases that may be caught from contact with someone who has the disease. I must immediately make it plain that there is no evidence at all that MS is catching or that it can be passed on by any form of contact. The curious pattern of MS in the relatively isolated Faeroe Islands has been cited as evidence of natural transmission of MS. Here there was a considerable increase in new cases between the years 1944 and 1960 and an attempt has been made to link this with the only notable change in environment in the islands in recent years, the presence of British troops during the Second World War. It is difficult to believe in the transmission of a hypothetical virus from healthy soldiers to the Faeroese, although this is not impossible. There is certainly nothing to suggest that those with MS contracted it from British soldiers with the disease. If MS was transmitted in this way an increased incidence in the spouses of those with the disease would certainly be expected but it is no higher than would be expected by chance. It is necessary to emphasize this because after every broadcast programme in which the theory of infection is discussed I find that misunderstanding can lead to people with MS being ostracized for fear that they will infect neighbours' children. There is no basis for this whatsoever.

It is particularly in the reporting of infective agents as the cause of MS that hope has so often been raised and almost equally often bitterly disappointed. Many of the earlier claims were in the relative infancy of bacteriology but on at least one occasion a claim, originally made in good faith, was eventually supported by fraudulent evidence. The exposure naturally had a most devastating effect on the eminent supporters of the project to make a protective vaccine from the supposedly responsible micro-organism. So frequent and so circumstantial have been the claims that those experienced in the field are now apt to greet with weary cynicism each new announcement for they know that even the most confident claims are hardly ever confirmed by other research workers. Some of the more important recent findings must be mentioned, particularly those still under investigation. As many of these are concerned with the possibility of virus infection something must be said about these micro-organisms by way of preliminary explanation.

Infectious diseases are caused by the invasion of the body by minute forms of living organisms, of which the most common are bacteria and viruses. Bacteria exist virtually everywhere, particularly in the soil, and the great majority of species live and multiply without ever invading man or any other living creature. Others exist harmlessly in the content of our intestines. Those that cause diseases can nearly always be easily identified, as bacteria can be seen under an ordinary microscope, particularly when stained by appropriate dyes. They can also be grown in suitable material, usually something resembling soup or jelly. The presence of invading bacteria can also often be inferred from the antibodies against them that are produced by their involuntary host.

Viral infection   Viruses are different in many ways. In the first place they are much smaller and even the largest of them cannot be seen under an ordinary microscope. They can be photographed under an electron microscope (EM) but this is very different from the intensive microscopic hunt that can be done when looking for bacteria. EM photographs of viruses do not at first sight suggest any form of living organism, as most viruses when 'seen' in this way look more like crystals or some other form of inanimate object. They are, however, alive in the sense that they can reproduce themselves by simple replication. Viruses can exist and remain infective outside the body but they can only multiply within living cells. Compared with bacteria, therefore, they are smaller, simpler forms of life and, most importantly in the context of MS research, much harder to find. Viruses induce antibodies in the same way as do bacteria but there is no possibility of growing them in the laboratory in the sort of broth and gelatine favoured by bacteria. Some forms of virus can be induced to infect living cells in tissue culture or in the embryo in a fertile hen's egg. It is quite likely that certain viruses can exist in forms different from those that can be recognized in EM pictures and much remains mysterious about their mode of existence in the body. Difficulties of identification are such that it was only in recent years that the virus of such a well-known disease as German measles or rubella was actually isolated. The difficulties inherent in such research in MS are indeed formidable.

One possibility still under investigation is that the infective agent might be a familiar virus acting in an abnormal or unusual way. A hint that this might be so is the finding that people with MS, on average, have the common childhood infections at a comparatively late age. There has been much interest in the measles virus. The first hint that measles might be involved came from studies of antibodies to common viruses in the blood of MS patients compared with the general population. There is now a considerable number of reports showing that the concentration of antibodies to measles is higher than expected in the MS patients. The difference is not great and is only detectable when results are taken from quite large groups of subjects, so this finding cannot be used as a diagnostic test for MS. There have been a few reports of increased antibodies to other viruses but these are much less consistent. What can this mean? Antibodies are formed during acute infections such as measles as part of the body's defences—an immune reaction. Usually when the infection has been overcome the level of antibodies falls, although often not as low as in subjects who have never been invaded by the particular virus. A persistently raised level is a hint that infection may also be persistent and that active virus might still be present.

It is now known that the measles virus can indeed persist within the central nervous system, although the disease in which this has been recognized is not MS but a very rare form of chronic inflammation of the brain (encephalitis) that affects children. These children have all had measles, often at an unusually early age, and only several years later do the progressive symptoms appear. The pathology does not closely resemble that of MS and this is not a primary demyelinating disease. Antibodies to measles are enormously increased in both the blood and cerebrospinal fluid and the actual measles virus in the brain can be shown by special staining methods. Why measles, the familiar, unpleasant, but normally essentially harmless infection of childhood, should occasionally behave in this way is unknown, but the important fact is that the virus persists silently in the brain for a latent period of some years before causing encephalitis. Perhaps if it persisted into adult life the result might not be encephalitis but MS, or so the argument has gone. A possible reason for such persistence might be some defect in the body's defences to measles, thus allowing the virus to persist in some form without being destroyed. There is no clinical evidence that patients with MS react differently to measles from anyone else and it is quite possible for an adult with MS who has escaped measles in childhood to have a typical attack of the disease. There is some evidence from specific laboratory tests that the immune reaction to the measles virus is defective in patients with MS but it now seems likely that this test is less reliable than was at first thought.

Much additional evidence of a highly technical nature has been found, suggesting that antibodies to measles are actually manufactured in the brain in MS and appear in the cerebro-spinal fluid in the increased immunoglobulin fraction of the proteins mentioned in Chapter 5. All this is, however, inference and the final step of demonstrating the measles virus itself in the central nervous system has not been achieved. Another report suggested the possibility of a different but related infective agent. Small scale studies showed that people with MS have closer contact with domestic cats and dogs than those who do not have the disease. This study has not so far been carried back into childhood but has related to the 10 years before the onset of the disease. There are obvious difficulties in obtaining such facts and they may not turn out to be correct, so there is certainly no reason for banishing the pet from the house. In this context it is significant that cats and dogs do not get measles, although the distemper virus closely resembles that of measles. Carefully controlled studies, however, comparing people with MS with unaffected people of the same age and sex, have shown no difference in the pattern of contact with domestic animals.

Another commonly encountered virus has recently come under suspicion that causing glandular fever, known as the Epstein–Barr virus. Infection with this virus is almost universal in adolescence and naturally most people with MS can be shown to have been infected in the past. There is a suggestion that people who have transient symptoms of involvement of the nervous system during a recognized attack of glandular fever might be more prone to subsequent MS and this possibility is being explored at present.

In tropical countries where MS is rare, particularly in the Caribbean, a progressive disease of the nervous system, tropical spastic paraplegia, causing severe difficulty in walking, has long been known. This has recently been shown to be due to infection with a retrovirus. These viruses are particularly difficult to detect as they may become latent or hidden in the chromosomes of the host. The AIDS virus, HIV, also belongs to this group. There have been claims that a different retrovirus could cause MS. This is extremely difficult to investigate but the evidence is not convincing.

Non-viral infection Infective agents other than viruses have come under suspicion. Ever since 1936 it has been known that the naturally occurring disease of sheep known as scrapie could be transmitted artificially to other animals, and that the transmissible agent had unusual properties, unlike those of a conventional virus, in particular being invisible and very hard to destroy. Much later it was shown that a disease of the brain occurring in certain tribes in New Guinea and known locally as kuru could be transmitted in the laboratory in the same way as scrapie. A very rare disease of world-wide distribution, called Creutzfeldt–Jakob disease after the doctors who first recognized it, has been shown to belong to the same group. Recent intense interest, and some alarm, has been aroused by the occurrence of a similar disease in cattle, apparently derived from adding ground-up sheep offal, presumably infected with scrapie, to the cattle feed. There is no evidence that this can be transmitted by eating beef. A number of attempts have been made to show that MS also belongs to this group of diseases but claims that material from a brain infected with MS had caused scrapie when injected into sheep were wrong and there is no reason to think that MS is in any way related, but the question is still often raised.

Less exotic infections have also been proposed as the cause of MS, including that common affliction, sinusitis, that accompanies every cold in the head. It was suggested that this could lead to invasion of the brain by organisms known as spirochaetes, which are frequent inhabitants of the nose, but this remains unproven and is an unlikely cause of MS. Certainly a proportion of MS relapses appear to follow mild infections but before most relapses there is no identifiable infection and a direct relationship is difficult to establish.

Genetic factors

The environmental factor therefore remains mysterious: what of the genetic influence? We have seen in Chapter 2 that MS is unduly common in close relatives of someone who has the disease and that the risk of twins both developing the disease is much higher with identical than non-identical pairs, the former necessarily sharing identical genes. It is probable that what might be handed down in families is not the disease itself but something in the makeup of the body that increases the risk of developing MS if exposed to the noxious agent in the environment. All the cells in all the tissues of any individual contain many antigenic substances in an individual pattern inherited through the parents' genes. They are antigenic because they are capable of stimulating the production of antibodies if introduced into the body of someone who does not naturally carry the same particular antigens. This, of course, was until recently a most unusual event, but kidney and other organ transplants are now common and it is the matching of these antigens as closely as possible between donor and recipient that is so important for the survival of the graft. This is not directly relevant to MS but the importance attached to these individual differences has drawn attention to the association of certain individual antigens belonging to the human leucocyte antigen (HLA) system and specific diseases. Among these is MS, where it has been reported that a higher proportion of individuals carry certain antigens than would be expected in the general population. Here again the proportions are not so abnormal as to be of any use in diagnosis and the possible implications are in relation to the functions of these HLA antigens in regulating the immune reactions of the body. It seems possible that certain combinations of antigens may be associated with a defect in these reactions, a defect that could permit the persistence in the body of a virus that would normally be destroyed or allow autoimmunity to develop.

All these theories are based on the idea that some poison or infection, deficiency, allergy, or inherent defect has a direct effect on the nervous system and causes MS. There is some evidence, however, that the immediate effect is not on the nervous system itself but on small blood vessels. The retina of the eye can be examined minutely during life and, by doing so, it has been found that in many people with MS there is patchy leakage from the retinal veins. Examination under the microscope, when this is possible, shows that such veins are surrounded by inflammation, as in an acute plaque in the nervous system. There is no myelin in the retina and these findings therefore show conclusively that inflammation around veins can occur in MS as the first event, not the result of break-down of myelin. This conclusion opens up a large field of future research.

A general theory of the cause of MS has received much support although it must be recognized that much of the evidence is flimsy and open to different interpretations. We may suppose that inborn defects in immune reactions permit the persistence in the nervous system of a virus, perhaps the measles virus, acquired in childhood. By direct attack by the virus or by stimulating autoimmunity to myelin, MS plaques are formed. The trigger that initiates the first attack and subsequent relapses remains unknown and this is but one of the many gaps in knowledge. The theory may be wrong, but there is continuing intense research activity directed to the detection and identification of an infective agent. How far this and other theories of causation have led to rational or effective treatment is considered in Chapter 7.

7 The treatment of multiple sclerosis

Many of those most intimately concerned with MS—those who have the disease, their relatives, and perhaps their medical attendants—will no doubt turn first to this chapter in the hope of learning of some new discovery. I must, therefore, at once make it plain that I do not believe that we have a cure for MS, but that this is no reason why treatment should not be attempted and indeed energetically pursued.

The treatment of MS is a subject that arouses intense and sometimes partisan emotions. The doctor has the problem of reconciling a desire to have an effective treatment with the objectivity that is absolutely necessary to a scientific discovery of such importance, at the same time avoiding the appearance of obtuse and rigid unwillingness to try unconventional remedies. As might be expected, not all succeed in this complex task. Those with MS and their families are naturally unfamiliar with the technicalities of assessing any therapeutic agent that is not an obvious immediate cure and with the peculiar difficulties posed by the fluctuating unpredictable course of MS. Anyone with the disease is not likely to await the result of a protracted trial before embarking on treatment for which *any* claims have been made. Indeed, no one would wish to discourage this unless the method was harmful to health or obviously a useless waste of money, but this is not the way to discover the cure.

The efficacy of treatment

Many people find it difficult to understand that there can be any problem in evaluating a proposed remedy for MS. Just hand it out and see if everyone gets better; if only it was so simple! To establish the efficacy of any form of treatment in medicine it is obviously necessary to compare the results in patients treated by the method under investigation with those in patients untreated or treated by some other means. It never fails to astonish me that doctors and scientists who have made notable contributions to many aspects of medicine are often blind to this self-evident truth when they approach MS. In other conditions this comparison sometimes does not present the slightest difficulty. For example, before the discovery of the antibiotic streptomycin, tuberculous meningitis was invariably fatal. To save even one patient's life was therefore a therapeutic triumph. The details of the regime of treatment were a matter for experiment, but there was never any doubt that it worked. Only slightly less obvious was the effect of the sulphonamide drugs on cerebrospinal fever, a form of acute meningitis. Here the high mortality rate and the incidence of dire complications among the survivors were only too well known, but some of those infected did come through unscathed. To treat a small series of patients was to be immediately and rightly convinced that sulphonamides were enormously superior to any treatment previously available. This conviction was, however, reached by comparing the results with those in a 'control' group, in this instance consisting of patients treated by other methods before the introduction of sulphonamides. The difference was so striking that, again, the issue was never in doubt.

Unfortunately the achievements of most forms of medical treatment fall far short of the dramatic, incontestable cure of previously intractable fatal disease, and consist more often of the partial alleviation of symptoms, the prevention of complications, and the prolongation of life in chronic disease. Here the comparison with the control group, a mere formality in the examples given above, assumes great importance and any apparent benefit in the treated group must not be described as 'striking' but in terms of significance—statistical significance. The difference between two sets of observations may be due to the influence of some discernible factor, in this instance the treatment, or to chance. Statistical methods can never totally eliminate the possibility of a chance result but can state the odds against it. Odds of $100 : 1$ or $1000 : 1$ against are clearly more

'significant' than 5 : 1 or 20 : 1 but significance must not be confused with *meaning*, which depends on many factors, not least
the relevance of the figures on which the calculation is based. If
these are incorrect or are not truly related to the outcome of the
treatment, then 'significance' becomes meaningless and mis-
leading.

The natural history of MS, described in earlier chapters, sets
many pitfalls for the unwary investigator. As an obvious
example, to give the favoured remedy at the height of a relapse
is to achieve what in most diseases would be an astonishing
success as the great majority of patients would recover or quickly
improve, but no conclusion at all can be drawn as to the value of
the treatment because recovery would have occurred naturally.
Similarly, a patient on continuous treatment who has no relapse
for five years would have reason to feel pleased, but not necessarily with the treatment, as this also could well be the natural
course. In the assessment of any form of treatment of MS the
most stringent precautions must be taken to obviate the effects
of chance, enthusiasm, prejudice, ignorance, incompetence,
and fraud. Control results recorded previously (and perfectly
adequate in demonstrating the revolution in treatment of meningitis), are not acceptable in MS, where new treatment must be
assessed against the course of untreated patients observed
during the same period of time in the same way at the same
centre. No ethical problem arises as the untreated group is not
deprived of any known benefit. At once, however, a new difficulty is encountered, that of *selection*. A trial in which all severe
cases were put in the untreated group would clearly be worthless, but much more subtle unconscious selection of patients by
the investigator can invalidate results. It is perfectly legitimate
to exclude certain categories of patients, perhaps those with
progressive disease or those with optic neuritis alone, but once
the criteria are established all patients who fulfil the conditions,
and who agree, must be admitted to the trial. They must then be
allocated to the treated or control groups at random, that is to
say, by some previously defined method, such as drawing a
card, in which chance is the only factor involved. This is the
basis of the randomized controlled trial.

A disadvantage of this method of assessment soon becomes apparent in practice. Although randomization ensures that 'bad' cases are not deliberately or unconsciously allocated to the untreated control group it does not by itself guarantee that the two groups will be properly matched with regard to any factor thought likely to be important—age, sex, severity of disease, and a host of others. This can only be overcome by using large numbers, when the laws of chance will *usually* ensure that the two groups are evenly balanced in all important respects. The larger the number of subjects the more likely this is to be so. The extreme variability of the course of MS is an additional reason for large numbers to be included, as results could readily be biased by an undue number of benign cases in either group.

The next problem is that of assessing the results, and here we encounter the problems of prejudice and of the placebo effect, the well-known benefits derived from a medicine without active ingredients and given only to please the recipient. Investigators will wish to see their methods of treatment proved successful or, if they are examining a treatment of which they disapprove, unsuccessful. Patients want to get better. There is a natural tendency to *feel* better if great interest is suddenly taken in one's previously perhaps relatively neglected condition by doctors enthusiastic about their new, impressive treatment. In addition to the possible benefits, the ill effects of treatment must also be assessed. The most alarming side-effects are quite often reported by people who prove to have been taking inert dummy tablets of chalk. All this requires the most careful planning before the trial is begun, but all will be wasted unless the investigation can be conducted *blind*. This means that neither the investigators nor the subjects know whether they are receiving the new treatment. The code concealing the allocation to the different groups is broken only after a predetermined large number of patients have been treated for an adequate period, so some safeguards must be incorporated to detect a harmful effect from treatment. A fully double-blind randomized controlled trial is often difficult or impossible to achieve and other methods of assessment may sometimes be unavoidable or at least acceptable but only with great reluctance in MS. There is no difficulty in finding enough people eager to enter a trial and willing to accept the chance that they might be taking dummy tablets for years. The problems of exactly what one is hoping to treat and how the results can be measured are quite another matter. The lesser aim is to reduce existing disability, either by diminishing the severity or duration of relapse or by alleviating chronic symptoms. The ultimate goal is, of course, complete cure, but how is this to be recognized when it is achieved? It is most unlikely that any form of treatment can be found that will reverse all the effects of long-standing disabling MS, as by this time there has certainly been some irreversible axonal degeneration. That is not to say that improvement could not be obtained, but a complete cure in the sense of a return to normal seems unattainable. A rational measurement of the effect of treatment designed to cure MS is the number of relapses, for these must surely be taken as evidence of activity of the disease.

Having decided this, the investigator determined to examine a definitive effect of any form of treatment on MS is still faced with problems. If relapses are to be counted they must be defined. When new symptoms and signs appear rapidly there is no difficulty in recognizing a relapse, but is an increase in already existing weakness or numbness also a relapse? Sometimes this is obviously so—for example, when a weak but serviceable leg rapidly becomes unable to bear weight in walking—but such examples can shade imperceptibly into a reported slight increase in weakness for a few days. Is this a relapse, a natural variation, a reversible effect of fatigue, or merely a subjective impression not based on any real change? The problem of recognizing a relapse, even when the new or increased symptoms are present when seen by a doctor, also emphasizes the importance of trying to measure the degree of disability. The results of examining the nervous system can be recorded at each visit but may be difficult to interpret in terms of significant change. A number of schemes have been proposed for recording the abnormalities in strength, co-ordination, vision, bladder control, and many other functions and for concocting a total score or disability rating. These methods are usually extremely time-consuming, which would not matter if they were informative, but unfortunately the scoring methods are either too sensitive, resulting in minute changes being recorded, or too coarse, so that mild but indisputable relapses hardly affect the record. All methods are highly susceptible to error or influence by the observer. There is a serious need for simple and more objective methods of assessment.

None of these difficulties would matter in the least if a really effective treatment was under trial, as this would reveal itself by the abolition of relapse, but as the usual rate of relapse is no more than once a year, about two years would be needed before the investigators broke the code of the blind trial and discovered the freedom from relapse of the treated group.

At the risk of repetition, I must emphasize the rational and, I believe, eventually productive approach to the treatment of MS. It is permissible and indeed useful to conduct a pilot trial of any form of treatment in perhaps a dozen subjects and to form an opinion on whether it should be abandoned as unavailing or harmful, or pursued as being of possible value. It is most certainly not permissible to advocate strongly any form of treatment on purely theoretical grounds or because a few people appear to have benefited. Those who have read the earlier chapters will be aware of the frailty of theories in MS and will know that the natural history of the disease in the early stages is of improvement after relapse. If, after anxious deliberation and preliminary trial, it is thought that a method of treatment is worthy of further exploration, the trial must approximate as closely as possible to the randomized blind controlled method outlined above. This is not to be undertaken lightly. The trial of continuous adrenocorticotrophic hormone (ACTH) therapy involved three large centres in Manchester, Leeds, and Belfast, 200 subjects and engaged the energies of several full-time research workers for 3 years, to show eventually that it was ineffective. Where blind assessment is impossible because of the nature of the treatment, controls must nevertheless be used. This is not to say that affected individuals should not try out any method that appears remotely promising, regardless of the results of trials—I would certainly do the same. I do not, however, think it is justifiable for anyone with pretensions or aspirations to the scientific method that can alone solve this problem to promote a form of treatment simply because it seems a good idea.

Fraud

Both the desperate need for treatment and the prolonged fluctuating course of the disease present openings for fraud, by which I mean treatment known to be worthless offered for financial gain. This opportunity for enrichment has only rarely been seized and even the most apparently bizarre forms of therapy have almost certainly been fervently believed in by their proponents. This sometimes demands a remarkable talent for self-deception, a commodity seldom in short supply. Patients should certainly not disburse large sums of money for supposed treatment without seeking advice, most helpfully from their national MS society.

Current treatment ideas

A number of different forms of treatment, curative or intended to improve function, are at present under review. Some of these are based on theories derived from the strange facts of the natural history and occurrence of MS. Others are the extension of accidental observations and yet others are simply based on what are hoped to be good ideas. In 1982 the International Federation of MS Societies published a loose-leaf book on *Therapeutic claims in MS*, in which over 70 forms of treatment of recent or current interest were briefly described and discussed.

Steroids

The word 'steroid' is often used rather loosely to include the different forms of cortisone and also adrenocorticotrophic hormone (ACTH). This latter substance does not belong to the chemical group of substances known as steroids but is a natural secretion of the pituitary gland, and stimulates the production of steroids, including cortisone, by the adrenal gland. A synthetic form of ACTH is also available, known under the trade of Synacthen. Cortisone itself is not now used in treatment, except simply to replace the secretions of the adrenal glands if these are destroyed. The usual preparations encountered in the context of MS are prednisolone and prednisone and, more rarely, dexamethasone. There are only minor differences in the action of these substances, probably of no importance. Steroid or cortisone treatment may cover any of these methods.

The initial use of cortisone and ACTH in MS was not based on any theory of how they might act on the disease but was undertaken simply on the grounds that here was a powerful form of treatment that had recently been shown to have unexpected results in a variety of hitherto intractable diseases, and it was natural to try it in MS. A further lead was that ACTH had been tried in post-infective encephalomyelitis, a demyelinating disease described in Chapter 6, and had seemed to induce an increased recovery rate. However tempting it was to use this treatment, all the difficulties of showing any effect remained, because steroids and ACTH did not produce immediate remission in chronic disease. Controlled trials have, however, been conducted and there is reasonably good evidence that a course of ACTH will speed recovery from relapse. In most centres, however, intravenous methyl prednisolone is now the preferred treatment for acute relapse and the form of ACTH previously used is no longer generally available.

Not every relapse needs treatment and many neurologists would not use steroids for optic neuritis in one eye or for symptoms such as numbness or pins and needles. Intravenous steroids do not actually increase the degree of improvement after relapse but there is no doubt that recovery is speeded up. A sharp attack of MS, perhaps with severe weakness, is frightening and rapid improvement is certainly welcome.

The technique involves the slow infusion over some hours into a vein of a dilute solution of methylprednisolone daily for from 3 to 5 days. Often, this course of treatment can be given as a hospital out-patient. Improvement is sometimes remarkably rapid and can only be the result of the immediate reduction of inflammation and swelling that can be seen by MRI. Side-effects are unusual. A nasty taste in the mouth is common but fleeting. Steroids may induce undue cheerfulness, unfortunately some-times followed by brief depression. The unpleasant acne and weight gain that were common with ACTH treatment are not seen unless steroids are given by mouth for some weeks after the intravenous course. This is sometimes recommended but I doubt if it does any good and the risk of side-effects is much increased. Unfortunately this advance in treatment of acute relapse is not effective in chronic disease, although often tried.

Steroid therapy should not be taken continuously for a long period because there is no evidence that it does any good. Some people with MS may become, in a way, dependent on prednis-olone in that, while the treatment does not appear to bring any relief, attempts to stop it are followed by an increase in the symptoms, only reversed by restoring the drug.

Immunosuppression

The main endeavour in the treatment of MS has been directed to suppression of the immune reactions of the body. The reason behind these attempts, it will be remembered, is the theory that autoimmunity to myelin is responsible, at least in part, for the damage to the nervous system caused by MS. If the body could be prevented from destroying its own myelin, relapses of the disease would stop, or so the theory goes. A number of drugs are used in conditions where it is necessary to suppress immune reactions, as, for example, in patients who have received a transplanted kidney or heart. As might be expected, all the drugs have undesirable side-effects and in high doses there are some risks of suppressing the normal reaction to infection.

Many of the processes of immunity are based on the action of a type of white blood cell, the lymphocyte, that we have already encountered in the earliest stages of the formation of the MS plaque. Full immunosuppression demands the removal of as many lymphocytes as possible, and there have been trials of highly elaborate combined forms of treatment designed to do just this. Such treatment cannot be continued for long and certainly did not effect a cure. It was claimed that relapses were less frequent following the treatment but this is a famous trap. Relapses *naturally* occur less often as the disease progresses, irrespective of any treatment.

A number of powerful immunosuppressant drugs—cyclophosphamide, cyclosporin and azathioprine—have been used singly or in combination with steroids. Cyclophosphamide, given intravenously, is still popular in the USA, although little used elsewhere: cyclosporin seemed to be of some help, but only in severely toxic doses. Azathioprine has been extensively examined in prolonged trials. Not everyone can tolerate it as it may cause vomiting. As with any immunosuppressant drug, regular blood tests are needed. Although slight benefit has been claimed in some trials, other results were negative and I am not convinced that azathioprine should be used.

Another method of immunosuppression involved exposing the whole body (except the central nervous system) to X-rays, thus preventing the normal production of lymphocytes. This was thought to slow the progress of MS but later trials have not been successful.

COP 1 COP 1 is a short title for copolymer 1, a synthetic product deliberately engineered to protect animals from experimental allergic encephalomyelitis (EAE) (see Chapter 6) without risk of aggravating this laboratory-induced demyelinating disease. The obvious next step was to try the effect on MS, with some apprehension. Again some success was claimed, although far short of a cure, but enthusiasm has waned and COP 1 is not at present available, although further trials are planned.

Transfer factor

The other attack on MS through immune mechanisms has been based on quite different ideas. It will be recalled from Chapter 6 that people with MS may have a defect in the way they react to the measles virus, and possibly to other infective agents. This possibility is derived from the results of laboratory tests and not from any observed difference in the way measles affects those with MS. If the theory of persistent infection is true then a defect in immune mechanisms that prevents the infection being overcome in the normal way could well be an essential factor in causing the disease. It has been known for some years that immunity can be transferred from one living creature to another by injecting an extract of white blood cells containing an ill-defined substance simply known as 'transfer factor'. Human transfer factor can be prepared and has been used in the treatment of small numbers of patients with MS with the aim of restoring normal immune reactions.

It is relatively easy to do satisfactory trials with transfer factor because all that is needed is a single injection once a month, producing no side-effects. The first trials were continued for a year and no benefit was seen. A more extensive trial in Australia was continued for two years and at the end of this period the treated patients were doing rather better than those given a blank injection. The extent of the benefit amounted to slowing progression of the disease and there was no question of cure, but obviously there were encouraging grounds for continuing the treatment. Unfortunately, benefit was not maintained on longer follow-up.

Antiviral treatment

If MS is possibly, or even probably, caused in some way by persistent virus infection, the most logical approach to treatment would be to kill the virus. Unfortunately the number of effective antiviral agents is very small and their range as regards the type of virus they can destroy is limited. There is so far nothing in this field in any way approaching the antibiotics that have revolutionized treatment of bacterial infections. Naturally attempts have been made to use what antiviral agents are available, although it must be confessed these have not been remarkable for their vigour. This is understandable, as these drugs act by interfering with the chemistry of the virus, which does not differ greatly from that of the normal cells of the body. Toxic effects are numerous and no benefits have been reported.

Interferon is not a single substance but exists in many forms with differing actions against viral infection and on the immune system and is a natural product of the body. Beta-interferon has been used in treatment of MS, being given by lumbar puncture as it was not thought to get through the blood–brain barrier when given by any other route. As with so many other forms of treatment the original claims were favourable but did not stand up to critical evaluation. A trial of beta-interferon given by other routes is in progress but I do not believe that many hopes are pinned on the result. Gamma-interferon appeared to make MS worse and was hastily abandoned.

Diet

All the treatments so far described have required, at the very least, close medical supervision, or at the most, highly sophisticated hospital facilities. The most widely used forms of treatment, however, are in a quite different category, as they are practised at home with no serious fear of harm and little need for detailed advice from the doctor. Two of these popular forms of treatment are concerned with diet.

The gluten-free diet in the treatment of MS is not based on any theoretical considerations, but is none the worse for that as we have seen that theories have so often proved sterile. Gluten is a component of wheat germ and is undoubtedly harmful in a particular disease of the gut known as coeliac disease. In this condition, gluten affects the lining of the gut so that many essential constituents of food, particularly fat, are not properly absorbed. This naturally has a most adverse effect on growth in children or on the general health of the adult, but complications involving the nervous system are rare. At any rate, gluten was known to be a potentially harmful constituent of the normal diet, although I must emphasize that it is harmful only to those with coeliac disease. It was probably on no stronger grounds than this that the gluten-free diet was first tried in MS.

The initial, and indeed the only, published evidence of benefit is based on the results in a single person whose regime included, among other deprivations, a gluten-free diet. There is no reason to doubt that he had MS and that while on the regime his condition improved to an unusual degree. To anyone knowledge-able in the natural history of MS, and by this stage this should include the readers of this book, the course of the disease in a single case, however remarkable, should occasion no surprise and would certainly not cause extravagant hopes of treatment. Just as certainly, no possible line of treatment should be neg-lected, particularly if harmless. The diet is a little troublesome to follow but consists essentially of using gluten-free flour in those items of food where flour is used, and these are more numerous than the uninstructed person would at first imagine. Soups and gravy are thickened with flour, for example, and bread seems to be incorporated into the most unlikely dishes. Gluten-free flour is readily obtainable and can be used in cooking and baking. Un-fortunately the regime does not work. From my own observa-tions I have seen too many relapses in patients on an apparently rigid gluten-free diet and a pilot trial has confirmed that the rate of relapse is not affected. This extremely disappointing result does not, of course, throw any doubt on the integrity of the original observations—the vagaries of MS are sufficient to lead even the most experienced astray. I advise against this diet, which leads to loss of weight and ill health.

Unsaturated fatty acids I now come to a very controversial aspect of the treatment of MS, at least in Britain, that of unsaturated fatty acids. Fatty acids are a normal constituent of animal and vegetable oils and fats. The word 'unsaturated' means that some of the carbon atoms that make up the basis of the chemical formula are linked by double bonds. They are unsaturated in the sense that the bonds could link with other atoms without break-ing the essential structure of the fatty acid molecule. This is exactly what is done when liquid fats are converted into solids in the preparation of normal margarine. Polyunsaturated fatty acids (PUFAs) contain several double bonds. In general, liquid natural oils contain a high proportion of unsaturated fatty acids while fats that are solid at room temperature contain mostly saturated fatty acids.

A popular idea seems to have grown up that saturated fatty acids are bad and in some way unnatural while unsaturated and particularly polyunsaturated fatty acids are good and natural.

This is something of a misconception as both forms of fatty acid are equally natural but occur in different proportions in different natural products including ourselves. It is indeed possible that PUFAs are better for us, as they reduce the level of cholesterol in the blood and perhaps thereby reduce the risks of stroke or heart attack. It is also true that in rats certain PUFAs have been shown to be 'essential'. Animals deprived of fat in the diet eventually develop a deficiency disease that can only be relieved by giving the PUFAs linoleic, linolenic, or arachidonic acids, which are therefore essential for the well-being of the rat. Linoleic acid can be converted in the body into the other two acids and is therefore the most important. A deficiency disease resulting from lack of these fatty acids has not been positively identified in man and there is certainly nothing resembling such well-known vitamin-deficiency diseases as scurvy or beri-beri.

The chain of reasoning linking fatty acids with MS is of great interest. The theory that high prevalence of MS is causally associated with a high intake of animal fat and saturated fatty acids was mentioned in Chapter 6. The evidence for this is far from watertight. Certainly, communities in Norway living close together but with different diets seem to fit this pattern but the diets were not analysed in any great detail and no doubt the modes of life of these villages differed in other ways. It was also claimed that a diet low in animal fat was beneficial to those with MS, but readers will by now be familiar with the fallibility of such claims not backed by figures and careful controls. Other evidence that has been advanced is somewhat less convincing—such as the low incidence of new cases of MS in concentration camps where the diet was low in fats, and indeed in everything else, and the increased incidence after liberation. Even if all these and other similar observations had been reliably confirmed they would not prove that MS was due to a diet high in animal fat, but at least the idea was well worth exploring.

There is also a very good reason to suppose that some abnormality in the way the body handles fat might well be involved in MS because, after all, myelin contains a high proportion of fat. It has been shown, not surprisingly, that the chemical analysis of the fats in areas of brain containing plaques of MS is different from normal. Of greater interest was the finding that areas of brain in which no plaques were visible also had an altered chemical composition, in particular a low proportion of PUFAs as compared with saturated fatty acids. If true, this could mean that the fat, and therefore the myelin, was abnormally constituted throughout the central nervous system in those with MS. This is the basis for the interesting idea of a life-long inborn abnormality of the composition of myelin that could render it vulnerable to attack from environmental agents such as infections. This possibility received support from the finding that the level of the PUFA linoleic acid was abnormally low in the blood of those with MS and that the more severe the disease the lower the level. It is only fair to say that these findings have been challenged by other research workers, who have concluded that a reduction in linoleic acid in the blood is merely an indication of severe disease—any kind of severe disease. Further work needs to be done but there is regrettably more than a hint of that disappointment so familiar to those who work with MS—the failure to confirm apparently highly significant findings.

There are indeed many reasons why a deficiency in PUFAs might contribute to MS. Fatty acids are an important component of the membrane that surrounds all cells and an imbalance between PUFAs and saturated acids could lead to vulnerability to invading organisms. PUFAs circulating in the bloodstream prevent the accumulation of the minute structures known as platelets, which are responsible for clotting of the blood. In certain circumstances these, together with red blood cells, conglomerate, or 'sludge', as it is elegantly known, and this process can block or damage small blood vessels. It will be remembered that MS plaques form around such small vessels. If people with MS do indeed have a low level of the PUFA linoleic acid in the blood it is not due to an inability to absorb this substance from the intestine, as feeding linoleic acid rapidly brings the blood level back to normal. There is therefore no link with the benefits claimed for the gluten-free diet, which improves absorption of fat in patients with coeliac disease. The exciting possibility remained that, however caused, a deficiency of linoleic acid or of other PUFAs might contribute to the breakdown of myelin and could be corrected by adding these fatty acids to the diet. A blind, controlled trial was therefore carried out in which the treated group had a daily ration of linoleic acid in an emulsion and the control group had a monounsaturated fatty acid, oleic acid. The trial continued for two years and was conducted in Belfast and King's College Hospital, London. The results, published in 1973, were unfortunately inconclusive. Relapses were not prevented but there was an indication that they were less severe in the treated group. The trial was well-conducted and would certainly have shown up a pronounced effect had it been present but numbers proved to be too small for proper statistical analysis of trends such as changes in the length or severity of relapse.

It may well be that PUFAs are used differently in the body in those with MS, but what part, if any, this plays in the causation of the disease is quite obscure. Experimentally it seems likely that linoleic acid has an immunosuppressant action, which could be responsible for any effect on the course of MS, if indeed this exists, rather than altering the composition of the fat within the central nervous system.

There is continuing interest in treatment with PUFAs, either in the form of sunflower seed oil or with the proprietary preparation Naudicelle. This is a capsule containing a mixture of PUFAs and other fatty acids. Particular emphasis is placed on the content of gamma-linoleic acid, which is readily converted to arachidonic acid in the body and therefore potentially of benefit to the formation of normal cell membranes. This acid is also involved in the formation in the body of the group of biologically very active but still rather mysterious substances known as prostaglandins. If there is anything in PUFA treatment of MS, the safest, most palatable, and economical method is to exclude fats that are solid at room temperature from the diet and to substitute soft margarine.

Rest/exercise

The third form of treatment that can be used by MS patients is the rest/exercise regime proposed by Professor Ritchie Russell.

As its name implies, this consists of set periods of quite violent exercise and complete rest during the day. I must confess that I have not been able to detect a scientific basis for this treatment but this would not be an obstacle to its working. It is claimed that those who faithfully carry out the programme will be relatively or perhaps entirely free from relapses, but this has not been assessed in any way at all resembling a controlled trial. Those fit enough to carry out vigorous exercise usually feel better for doing so but in my own experience it does not prevent relapse or continued deterioration.

Hyperbaric oxygen

The use of hyperbaric oxygen in the treatment of MS still has its advocates. 'Hyperbaric' means increased pressure. Breathing oxygen at twice the atmospheric pressure, or rather greater, has been used as a method of producing a high concentration of oxygen in the body when damage was threatened by lack of oxygen. This was particularly successful in coal gas poisoning but less so in other conditions where it was hoped it might be useful, and most of the hyperbaric oxygen chambers installed in hospitals fell out of use as coal gas was superseded by natural gas. Chambers in which high pressures can be obtained are in routine use in decompressing deep sea divers.

The original reason for trying hyperbaric oxygen in the treatment of MS was not, perhaps, very exciting. It had been found that exposure to oxygen under increased pressure would delay or prevent the onset of allergic demyelinating encephalitis in experimental animals, but many agents were already known to do this, including PUFA. Subsequently the use of hyperbaric oxygen has been linked to the controversial theory that MS plaques result from blockage of blood vessels, causing lack of oxygen.

Hyperbaric oxygen can be given in a pressure chamber large enough to hold a single person, into which oxygen is pumped at the required pressure. An alternative method is for the chamber to be filled with air under pressure and for oxygen to be breathed through a mask while in the chamber, resulting in

oxygen under similar pressure, and this is the method commonly used in MS.

The usual course of treatment consists of 90 minutes in the
chamber daily for five days a week for some six weeks, all these
figures being based on convenience rather than anything more
scientific. Nobody should undertake such treatment without
medical advice and, in particular, changes in pressure can have
unpleasant effects on blocked ears and sinuses. However, with
reasonable care, no harm should result.

The question of whether the treatment does any good originally ran into the usual difficulties. In large uncontrolled trials it
was claimed that most patients benefited, some substantially. In
an ingenious trial in which neither patient nor doctor knew
whether oxygen or air was being given under pressure, those
having oxygen did rather better. Further detailed trials in many
countries have failed to show any significant benefit. This is
naturally very disappointing to those who enthusiastically
adopted the regime, but probably no form of treatment of MS
has been examined so carefully and the result can scarcely be
challenged. I do not dissuade people from attempting this
treatment, but I have never seen it do any good.

Unconventional methods

Dismayed by the obvious failure of conventional medicine,
many have naturally turned to other forms of treatment; among
them herbs, snake venom, rays, manipulation, and acupunc-
ture. It is extremely improbable that any of these forms of
treatment has any fundamental effect on the underlying disease
process but temporary improvement in morale is frequent and
worthwhile, if not bought at too high a price. Finally, it is not
the doctor's place to deter anyone from seeking help from faith-
healing or to pronounce on the possibility of miraculous cure.

Conclusion

In this chapter I have looked at methods of treatment designed
either to effect a cure or a reduction in severity of the disease

process or to have an effect on total disability. Treatments directed to specific symptoms will be considered in the next chapter. I began by saying that I did not believe we had a cure for MS but that this is certainly not for want of trying. Advances in treatment must depend on inspiration linked to detailed research in the laboratory, in the hospital, and at home. MS is bound to give rise to emotional responses, as nobody can be unmoved when they see a young person crippled by perhaps the third or fourth relapse. Such emotions can certainly provide the motive for research but must be abandoned when the results are to be assessed. The practice of personal advocacy of forms of treatment after uncontrolled trials has led to false hopes and bitter disappointments and should surely be abandoned.

8 *Practical points*

There are many matters of importance in everyday life on which those intimately concerned with MS need advice, among them the treatment and management of certain specific symptoms.

Spasticity

Spasticity has already been described in Chapter 3 and is the result of increased reflex activity induced by stretching the muscles, most importantly in the legs. It is common in MS because of the damage to the descending motor pathways in the spinal cord that normally control these reflexes. In walking the effect of spasticity is to hold the legs straight at the knees with the feet pointing downwards, resulting in a stiff and awkward gait and scraping of the toes on the ground. An advantage of the legs being held in this position is that they form efficient props, allowing the upright posture to be maintained. Spasticity of this degree in legs already weakened may be uncomfortable but often assists walking rather than impedes it. To abolish spasticity here may result in weak legs that can no longer be held straight or support the body's weight. Theoretically it should be possible to reduce the overactivity of the reflexes without producing weakness but after years of trial I have concluded that none of the numerous drugs that have been claimed to do just this is effective to the point of making it easier to walk.

Many people with moderate spasticity experience extensor spasms. These are apt to happen in bed at night or on waking in the morning. Both legs shoot out straight and for a brief period may be difficult or impossible to bend. These spasms are seldom painful but are somewhat alarming when they first occur. As they do not last more than a minute or so at first and are usually much more brief the degree of disability is equally slight and treatment is not required unless they are painful or extremely frequent. If extensor spasms are prolonged they can sometimes be immediately terminated by change in posture of the neck, particularly bending the chin down towards the chest.

A more important and certainly more distressing symptom is one that may appear later if spastic weakness progresses. The reflex contraction of the muscles that hold the spastic legs straight gives way to spasm in the opposing muscles that bend the leg at the hip and knee joints. These flexor spasms can occur during walking and result in falling but are more common in bed or sitting in a chair. They are much more apt to be painful than extensor spasms and when severe can make it almost impossible to find a comfortable position either sitting or lying. They are aggravated by any sore place on the legs or by infection in the bladder and may be greatly helped if these complications are treated successfully. One drug is often successful in controlling flexor spasms, although of much less use in other forms of spasticity. This is baclofen, which can be taken in gradually increasing doses until a worthwhile effect is reached. It is in no sense a cure; baclofen has a specific action on damping down abnormally active reflexes. The effect of giving baclofen by injection into the cerebrospinal fluid around the spinal cord has been investigated recently. Relief can be dramatic but the elaborate method is not free from complications and is not in general use.

In really severe cases of spasticity in the flexed position in bedridden subjects, more permanent measures are justified and useful and, when successful, they allow comfortable sitting in a chair and greatly ease nursing care. The method employed in a few centres is the injection of phenol in glycerine by lumbar puncture. This has a destructive effect on nerve fibres and the aim is to direct this to the nerve roots carrying impulses to and from the spinal cord. However, reflexes cannot be completely abolished without causing any other additional symptom and this method is only employed in people who are already severely disabled, and not in those still able to walk. Operations that reduce spasticity by cutting muscles or their nerve supply are used comparatively rarely in MS as the necessary period immobile in bed after the operation, even if this is kept to a minimum, has an adverse effect on subsequent mobility.

Tremor

If intention tremor, described in Chapter 4, is severely incapacitating it can sometimes be helped by applying lead weights in the form of wrist bands. These have the effect of reducing the tremor but naturally have the disadvantage of taxing the strength of weakened limbs.

Surprisingly, very severe tremor can sometimes be reduced or abolished by an operation on the brain. This involves making a small, very precisely placed area of destruction in one of the centres in the brain that control movement. The operation, although very skilled, is not a major procedure and can be very successful. There are, however, some risks and few people are sufficiently incapacitated by tremor to warrant this form of surgery.

Neuralgia

Trigeminal neuralgia and the other paroxysmal symptoms described in Chapter 4 respond in a remarkable way to the drug carbamazepine, sold under the trade name of Tegretol. Within half an hour of the first dose symptoms that had been occurring up to 80 times a day stop completely. Such an immediate response is rare enough in any disease and is certainly remarkable in MS. Treatment must be continued but usually a low dose without side-effects is successful. After a few weeks the dose can be reduced, and if symptoms do not return the drug is no longer needed. Trigeminal neuralgia can sometimes prove obstinate and eventually become resistant to treatment but can then be relieved by an injection into the nerve, which unfortunately also causes some loss of sensation on the face. Less destructive methods using radiofrequency waves are also successful. Tegretol does not have a beneficial effect on the other symptoms of MS, with the exception that the pins and needles produced by bending the head forward experienced by some patients can also be abolished. All these symptoms seem to derive from over-activity of certain elements of the nervous system, as opposed to the results of reduction of function, such as weakness and ataxia. It is my impression that these latter symptoms are, in fact, aggravated by Tegretol, although only while the drug is being taken and not as a persistent effect.

Incontinence

Failure of control over the bladder and bowel are among the most grievous results of spinal cord disease and are common in moderately advanced MS. The various degrees of this disability were described in Chapter 4. Urgency of the desire to pass water or, less commonly, to pass a motion, can often be helped by drugs. These act either directly on the muscle of the bladder or rectum or on their nerve supply. The best of these, terodiline (Micturin) unfortunately had to be withdrawn because it sometimes caused irregularity of the heart in elderly people who did not have MS. The latest introduction is oxybutinin (Ditropan) but a number of other drugs have very similar effects, including emepromium (Cetiprin) and propantheline (Probanthine). These measures may make life more tolerable but are not always helpful and many patients remain apprehensive if more than a short distance from a W.C. Limiting the amount of fluid drunk on specific occasions as, for example, on an outing from home, is uncomfortable but is not dangerous for short periods, and many find this preferable to constantly looking around for the nearest comfort station.

Getting up several times a night to pass water can be exhausting, particularly if the legs are weak. The pituitary gland makes a hormone that cuts down the amount of urine formed and some people find that taking this in the form of nose drops (desmopressin) at bedtime will see them through the night. A method of management that many people have found extremely helpful is self-catheterization. A catheter is a tube of silicon-treated rubber that can be passed into the bladder through the natural passage, allowing the bladder to be completely emptied. Some obvious problems arise. Steady hands are essential and training is also necessary. The fear of introducing infection into the bladder seems to have been exaggerated, and cleanliness a good deal short of the sterile procedures of the operating theatre seems to be perfectly satisfactory.

At a more advanced stage, incontinence of urine cannot be influenced at all by drug treatment and management consists of minimizing the inconvenience. This is far easier in the male because the penis can be fitted into the opening of a rubber urinal that can be strapped to the leg and, with perseverance, this method will prevent soiling of the clothes in the daytime. This device cannot be worn at night or when lying down as it simply overflows but this can be overcome by a rubber contraceptive condom with the end cut off connected to a tube leading to a receptacle. There may be difficulties in fixing these devices but these can be overcome by ingenuity and sometimes with special adhesives. More difficult to deal with is skin sensitivity to rubber or adhesive plaster.

Women are at a serious anatomical disadvantage and no efficient urinal has yet been invented. The best that can be done is to adopt a routine with absorbent padding and waterproof pants. This solution is obviously far from ideal and to a normally fastidious woman urinary incontinence can be emotionally most distressing. Great efforts have been made to find an alternative method. There seems to be an increasing tendency to use a catheter for incontinence, retained in the bladder by some device such as a small balloon that can be distended once the catheter is in place. This certainly prevents incontinence as the urine can be drained away as it forms or intermittently, but at a cost. A catheter may be essential if there is *retention* of urine; that is to say if the bladder becomes distended because urine cannot be passed at all. This is usually temporary and the catheter is withdrawn. Incontinence is unfortunately often permanent and a permanent catheter, however carefully maintained and changed, always leads to infection of the bladder, with the risk of spread to the kidneys or the bloodstream. This risk is not acceptable if disability is otherwise not severe. In bedridden people a balance has to be struck between the risk of urinary infection and of bedsores resulting from perpetual soaking of the skin with urine. In these circumstances a catheter is preferable.

Other solutions have been tried. The urine has been discharged through an artificially constructed bladder to the front of the abdomen, where it is relatively easy to fix collecting bags. This works less well than was hoped because of unforeseen complications. Electrical devices designed to stimulate normal bladder reflexes have not yet been perfected. Urinary incontinence, particularly in women, remains a distressing disability.

Loss of control of the bowel is often a less serious problem. Constipation is common if there is severe involvement of the spinal cord. Constipation in itself does not give rise to the events that might be expected from laxative advertisements and, apart from discomfort, is harmless. It is certainly more convenient to establish a routine but aperients should not be taken as these often cause incontinence of bowel movements. A small enema or suppositories, either of simple glycerine or containing some agent such as the effective Dulcolax, are best but any idea that a daily motion is essential for clean living should be abandoned. Twice a week is ample.

Bed sores

Bed sores result from continuous pressure temporarily obliterating the small blood vessels that carry oxygen and other nutriments to the skin. In health we seldom keep still for long, even when asleep in bed, and these frequent changes in posture prevent any area of skin from being deprived of blood for more than a brief period. In anyone who lies or sits immobile for more than a few hours, the skin, compressed by the weight of the body against a hard surface, may die for lack of oxygen. If pressure is maintained the deeper tissues, fat, and muscle, are also destroyed and in the days before this was understood paraplegic patients would develop horrifying sores in which the bones were exposed. These will be painless if there is loss of sensation in the area but are highly dangerous as sites where infection can gain access and from which essential nutriments, particularly protein, can drain away.

The message is plain. Anyone who cannot move or who cannot feel that harmful pressure is building up must be moved passively every two hours. I have often been astonished at the skill, devotion, and success with which this arduous regime is maintained in many homes—and occasionally ashamed at its breakdown in hospital wards not alert to the problems of the disabled. Bed sores, once formed, are difficult to heal. Further pressure must be avoided at all costs and infection must be cleared but, after many experiments, I do not think that any particular form of dressing has notable advantages. Large intractable sores may require skin grafting and often then heal well under expert care.

In ideal conditions bedsores can be completely prevented by turning, sheepskins to lie on, and ripple beds, but overweight and incontinence may obviously present difficult problems, and conditions are by no means always ideal.

Sex

MS does not directly interfere with sexual function in women but weakness, spasticity, and reflex spasms may cause mechanical difficulties in intercourse. Vaginal secretions may dry up and can be replaced by lubricating jelly. Blunting of normal sensation unfortunately cannot be helped. Impotence in men can be caused by spinal cord disease but the degree of variation is remarkable. In some men impotence is an early symptom of MS but others with moderately severe disease retain potency. Impotence can, of course, arise from psychological causes that could well respond to treatment, and advice should certainly be sought. Desire is not diminished but what is lost is the ability to obtain or sustain an erection. Surgical measures have been devised for introducing artificial stiffening into the penis and some have found this satisfactory. It is not always easy to find a surgeon familiar with the technique. Within the last few years the technique of self-injection of papaverine directly into the penis has been found to be remarkably effective in the treatment of many forms of impotence, including that in MS. The technique must be learnt in a special clinic and adjusted to the smallest dose effective in producing an erection. There are occasional complications and it could not be claimed that this preliminary to making love is exactly romantic but it is a great deal better than nothing. Failure of the normal sexual relationship is an obvious source of stress in a young married couple. If it cannot be cured it is still far better that it should be discussed openly rather than concealed or regarded with shame. Mutual sexual stimulation short of full intercourse may provide at least a partial solution. Many doctors are curiously inhibited in giving advice on sexual matters, but fortunately the widely prevalent but unspoken idea that handicapped people do not have human needs is rapidly being dispelled.

Children

The question of heredity was discussed in Chapter 2. There remain the practical aspects of childbirth and rearing a family. Some 20 years ago MS was regarded as an absolute bar to having children on the grounds that relapse was commonly precipitated by pregnancy. This extreme view is no longer held. There is a relatively slightly increased risk of sustaining a relapse during the pregnancy year, that is to say, the nine months of the pregnancy, and especially so in the subsequent three months of the puerperium. On the other hand it is doubtful whether such relapses have any effect on the final outcome. I have known many young women who have deliberately taken the risk and have not regretted it. An enduring memory is of a pregnant girl with MS whose husband had just had a serious accident. We discussed the question of termination but her decision was: 'Nothing nice ever happens to us; let's have the baby'. I am glad to say that this at least turned out well.

A large family is obviously undesirable both because of the recurrent increased risk of relapse and of the difficulty of looking after the children if the disease proves to be severe. Similarly the economic aspects of rearing a family should be discussed should the breadwinner become disabled. These are personal decisions to be guided by informed advice.

Physiotherapy

I have included physiotherapy in this chapter as it must certainly be regarded as treatment of symptoms rather than curative. Modern physiotherapy no longer consists of massage and electric shocks but of exercise and retraining of the performance of movement. A skilled physiotherapist can contribute greatly to the recovery of a patient who has had a relapse of MS involving weakness of the legs. The contribution consists partly in instruction in making the best use of remaining functions and partly in the boost to morale resulting from the enthusiastic attention of someone who clearly knows what they are doing. I do not believe that physiotherapy actually alters the pathological process of MS in the slightest and physiotherapists would not claim that it does. Many of those who have MS have a great faith in physiotherapy but its value to someone with static or slowly progressive disease lies, I believe, solely in the effect on morale. I am naturally all in favour of spirits being raised in this way but physiotherapy departments are nearly always understaffed and those with MS who do not attend regularly for physiotherapy, and this is the majority, are not being deprived of some great benefit. Indeed, long ambulance rides to crowded departments for 20 minutes' exercise is more a recipe for exhaustion. People are often concerned as to how far they should exercise at home in carrying out what they have been taught by physiotherapists. Exercise to maintain mobility is obviously beneficial but most would believe that serious fatigue should be avoided. Walking aids are often used reluctantly because of the obvious indication of invalidism. A stout umbrella with a rubber tip is an acceptable substitute for a walking stick. Quadrupod sticks and walking frames greatly assist independence and emotional resistance to their use should be gently overcome when they prove necessary. Splints and calipers on the legs are seldom helpful. If the feet are strongly pointed downwards by spasticity it is tempting to try to pull them up with springs but these have to be so strong that the resulting weight of ironware is an added burden, besides being unsightly. Reluctance to use a wheelchair is often expressed on the grounds that this is a sign of 'giving in'. This is understandable. The advantages of a chair, when it does become necessary, are soon appreciated.

Occupational therapy is also of great value in teaching the partially disabled to make the most of their capabilities at work and particularly at home. A skilled assessment of the feasibility of alterations to the house is invaluable (see Plate 11), and this can often be obtained through hospital occupational therapy departments working in conjunction with local authorities.

Work

The person with MS should aim to keep at work. Numerous jobs are obviously impossible and there are others that are undesirable. Many factory jobs entail standing all day long at a bench or machine, tiring enough even if one's legs are strong. It is by no means certain that fatigue causes relapse but chronic fatigue is cause enough for feeling continually unwell. Many employers will do their utmost to find appropriate work and, if this is not available, workmates are remarkably accommodating. It is often getting to work that is the greater problem. It is not possible safely to control the pedals of a car with spastic legs, and hand controls are essential. Quite apart from the practicalities of work, continued mobility outside the home is of supreme importance in maintaining morale. The sense of confinement within four walls, dependent on others' kindness for outings in the car, is oppressive. Invalid cars for use on the high road have not been notably safe or mechanically sound, but have brought joy into the lives of many MS sufferers. If financial means can be raised there is an electrically propelled buggy available that can also provide the boon of at least partial independence. It is extremely important to maintain contact with people who are not disabled and not to accept isolation from the accustomed social round.

Surgical operations

It used to be thought that operations and anaesthetics were dangerous in MS and were apt to bring on relapse. It has been repeatedly shown, however, that the great majority of operations are not followed by any setback and necessary surgery should certainly be accepted without any such fears. On the quite unscientific idea of 'not rocking the boat' unnecessary, purely cosmetic surgery should probably be avoided.

The only form of anaesthetic that has been shown to do harm in MS is the spinal anaesthetic given by lumbar puncture and this should not be used. This is quite different from the epidural block often used during childbirth, which has not been found to be harmful. Dental extractions can be done under either local or general anaesthesia.

Inoculations

There were possible grounds for fearing that inoculations might aggravate MS but these have not proved to be justified. Smallpox vaccination was occasionally the cause of an acute and dangerous disease of the nervous system that in some ways resembled acute MS. I have not seen vaccination cause a relapse in anyone with MS but I am relieved that smallpox has been eradicated and that vaccination is no longer necessary.

There were also fears that influenza vaccine might carry similar dangers in MS, as an acute demyelinating disease of the central or peripheral nervous system can occasionally follow the use of this vaccine. This has been most carefully looked at in the USA, where there had been great anxiety following an increase in neurological disease caused by a certain influenza vaccine. No evidence was found that this vaccine did any harm in MS.

Depression

It might be thought natural that anyone with a chronic and, at least potentially, serious disease would feel depressed for much of the time. Fortunately this is not so in MS: and this statement is not based simply on the brave face that many people assume when seeing the doctor. Nevertheless, depression is rather more common than in people who do not have MS, and by depression I do not mean the transient gloom of Monday morning. Persistent low spirits, loss of appetite, and poor sleeping, especially with waking in the small hours full of gloomy and reproachful thoughts, are symptoms of a depressive *illness*, an illness that will very probably respond to specific treatment. So a smiling face and brave front, however admirable, should not be used to cover depression of this kind, for which help is needed and available.

Publications

There are many short books and pamphlets describing from personal experience how best to cope with physical and psychological problems of MS. Among these can be recommended *Learning to live with MS* by Robin Dowie, Robert Povey, and Gillian Whitley, available from the MS Society of Great Britain.

Miscellaneous

There is no evidence that smoking or drinking alcohol aggravates MS. Tolerance for alcohol may be reduced so that ordinary social doses may produce unexpected unsteadiness, but this is just a passing effect. In a very few people the nicotine in tobacco smoke may also increase unsteadiness and, in some, sensitivity to an increase in temperature may be so great that smoking a cigarette or drinking a cup of tea can cause blurred vision for a few minutes.

The contraceptive pill has no adverse effect on MS.

Home or hospital

Nearly everybody prefers their own home to a hospital bed. Those with MS may need hospital admission for investigation to establish the diagnosis and for care during acute relapses. In many homes it would clearly be impossible to provide suitable rest, nursing care, and the graduated return to activity needed during a relapse of any severity. Apart from these acute events there is an unfilled and often desperate need for residential care for the severely disabled. Not every home is equal to the exacting physical and mental strain of constant unremitting care. What is needed, and is so inadequately provided, is a combination of skill and kindness in premises less obviously 'clinical' than a hospital ward. All those concerned in any way with MS should lose no opportunity to press for the establishment of more such homes where those in need can be cared for, either temporarily to give the hard-stretched family a rest, or as a permanent refuge.

The doctor's role

The idea that it is the doctor's aim and duty to cure a patient's every ill does not survive long in practice. Apart from infections, injuries, and surgical emergencies, most diseases are 'incurable' in the sense that they cannot be completely eradicated, but nevertheless their effects can be alleviated by treatment. Even if, as in MS, treatment of symptoms is only partially successful, the doctor still has a part to play. To have a chronic disease of any kind, particularly a strange illness like MS, so difficult to explain to others, is to feel in some way set apart and isolated, or so I have often sensed in those who have consulted me. There is a need to talk to someone who knows and cares about those who have MS, and whether this be the general practitioner, the neurologist, or general physician is not important as long as the attributes of knowledge and concern are there.

There is one difficult aspect of a doctor's role that causes heart-searching and indecision; the classic question of 'should a doctor tell?'. Everyone must be treated as an individual but I have come to certain definite general conclusions. I do *not* tell anyone that I think they have MS after a single attack from which they have recovered, and this is for two reasons. First, no doctor is infallible and the diagnosis may be wrong. Second, if it is right, remission may still last for months, years, or even indefinitely, and on both counts it would be wrong to burden these years with fear. On the other hand, if you think you have MS you should ask the doctor and should not be put off by evasions such as 'a demyelinating disease like MS' or 'an obscure virus infection'. If, as now happens frequently, I am asked at this stage: 'Is it MS?' I say that this is one of the diagnoses I am considering, and I try to explain the difficulties of being more precise.

When I am certain of the diagnosis I always say so. I have often been urged by relatives not to do so on the grounds that this would cause panic or depression, but this does not happen. Not only are people braver than we think but they are also more intelligent and usually more than half suspect the diagnosis before the news is broken. Concealment of the truth from an adult who will have to live with it for 25 years or more is absurd. Moreover, it is distasteful to suspect that your doctor is telling lies and scarcely encouraging to believe that he or she has no idea what is wrong with you.

The MS Society

The MS Society is an almost totally admirable institution. Its intentions are to raise money for research and to improve the lot of those with MS by practical means and by the spread of information. People with MS should certainly join the local branch and, equally important, the uninvolved members of the public would find this a worthy object of their energetic support. The Society can provide sensible and accurate advice about proposed methods of treatment and about practical measures for the relief of disability. My only slight reservation is that some of those with MS do not like to attend meetings, as they will undoubtedly meet people with severe disability, and this can be frightening. This is an individual matter on which no general advice can be given. From personal observation of local branches many of the most severely disabled people who attend meetings may not have MS at all but quite different diseases of the nervous system, but I do not reveal this fact.

The addresses of the National Societies in English speaking countries are as follows:

Australia   34 Jackson St, Toorak, Victoria, 3142
Canada   Suite 820, 250 Bloor Street East, Toronto, Ontario, M4W 3P9
Great Britain   25 Effie Road, Fulham, London, SW6 1EE
New Zealand   PO Box 2627, Wellington
Republic of Ireland   2 Sandymount Green, Dublin 4
Republic of South Africa   295 Villiers Road, Walmer, Port Elizabeth, 6065
United States   733 Third Avenue, New York, N.Y. 10017
Zimbabwe   PO Box 8214, Causeway, Harare

9 *The future*

As mentioned in the preface to this book there is now a feeling of hopeful expectancy among those most involved in MS. To what extent is this justified, particularly in the face of the long tale of frustration that I have had to relate? The last few years have seen an enormous expansion of the application of sophisticated laboratory research methods to the problems of MS. The interpretation of the results is often difficult and subject to detailed understanding of the minutiae of the methods employed. Those not involved in a given field of research must accept at face value results published in reputable scientific journals, or await the experiments or opinions of other experts in the relevant techniques. Sophistication of laboratory methods does not, unfortunately, always lead to consistent results. Indeed, the more complex the procedure the greater the room for error or disagreement. The essential clue that will permit the trail of causation to be followed back to the point at which effective treatment can be applied is likely to be found in systematic research, although a shaft of genius illuminating the subject from a quite unexpected angle is also possible.

The search will continue for an infective agent, presumably a virus, although perhaps modified in some way that has so far allowed it to escape detection. The discovery of a virus that causes a disease does not mean that a cure is immediately available. If poliomyelitis again broke out in those countries from which it has been virtually eradicated we would be powerless to halt its effects as we have no means of killing the virus in the body. The very success of the poliomyelitis vaccination shows what can be achieved in virus control. Whether a vaccination programme could be launched against a disease that affects no more than 1 in 1000 people is problematical and would be a matter for anxious deliberation. All this depends on a successful outcome to the hunt, and techniques in present use have not yielded consistent results. New methods in virology may be needed. The possibility of some non-infective environmental agent, some poisonous substance, still exists but now seems less probable.

From time to time I am asked to take part in discussions on 'The Needs of the Patient with MS'. What is talked about at such meetings is certainly of great importance in everyday life and even now these practical matters are often badly neglected. However, nobody with MS has any doubt that the single over-powering 'need' is for effective treatment—a cure if possible or, if not, some way of preventing further attacks or deterioration.

Anyone who has read Chapter 7 on 'treatment' should be aware of the great difficulties involved in mounting a proper trial of any form of treatment—a trial that will end with a definite answer. The treatments described in that chapter are only a small fraction of those that have been tried, sometimes based on well-thought-out scientific theories and sometimes nothing more than a shot in the dark. Very few have been subjected to rigorous trial and probably the perfect trial of treatment in MS has never been carried out.

A full-scale, double-blind, placebo-controlled trial of treatment of MS is extremely arduous both for those receiving and those giving the treatment. It is also extremely expensive, may last for several years, and involves a great many people. A method of achieving a comparatively quick result in a small group of people would be an enormous advance. Such a method may be at hand. MRI scanning, even in people with MS who are free from relapse, shows that the disease remains active, as frequent, fresh abnormalities appear on scans repeated at quite short intervals. If routine scanning is combined with injection of an 'enhancing' agent the new lesions have a characteristic appearance. The agent used, gadolinium, does not pass through the normal blood–brain barrier but, when this is broken, it will enter the nervous system and will be shown on the scan. In each new lesion a small area of such enhancement by gadolinium is surrounded by a large area that is abnormal but that does not enhance. After a few weeks the central enhancement is no longer present and the wider area shrinks. This pattern has been interpreted, surely correctly, as showing breakdown of the blood–brain barrier with a small area of inflammation surrounded by swelling. In serial scans these events, showing disease activity, occur far more frequently than relapses causing symptoms. The hope is that serial enhanced scans in people receiving a treatment under trial would very quickly show whether the disease process was still active or had been halted. This may sound a simple procedure but most meticulous technique is essential. This exciting prospect is very largely due to the work of Professor W.I. MacDonald and his team at the National Hospital for Neurology and Neurosurgery in London, supported by the MS Society.

It will be a great achievement to have an objective method of assessing treatment quickly, but are there methods of treatment worth trying?

Immunosuppression, despite earlier disappointments, remains an important prospect. Methods already tried have suppressed immunity in a totally unselective way. One problem is that if autoimmunity is indeed the key, we do not precisely know the antigen; that is to say the exact component of the nervous system that is being rejected. Myelin, or some fraction of myelin, is an obvious candidate, but this has not been conclusively proven, and treatments based on this assumption have not been fruitful. Trials of immunosuppression are, however, now being more sharply directed, using monoclonal antibodies to specific types of lymphocyte, thought to be involved in MS lesions, rather than simply destroying them all.

Another aspect of immunosuppression is that none of the agents that have been used in MS actually penetrate the blood–brain barrier to a significant extent. Perhaps it is not necessary to do so but the development of a drug that was known to reach the site of the disease would be an interesting project.

Research is also turning to the blood vessels of the nervous system and the means by which blood cells first adhere to the wall of the vessel and then pass through. We have seen how important a step this is in the formation of an MS plaque.

Attention is also being paid to the question of repair. Remyelination is now accepted as probable in MS but eventually fails. The cells that make the myelin sheaths, the oligodendrocytes, are formed from more primitive cells, but little is known of how this could be encouraged to begin the repair process. Long-term research has begun on the prospect of injecting oligodendrocytes, or their precursors, into the nervous system in the hope that they might survive and carry out their normal function of myelination.

One factor that may prevent repair in MS is the scarring—the sclerosis—that forms in chronic plaques. Methods of preventing this are now being explored.

It is to be hoped that in all this press of basic laboratory science the welfare of people with MS will be kept well in the foreground with the aim of alleviation of symptoms while prevention and cure are awaited.

People with MS often ask whether there have been recent advances in research and whether a cure is just around the corner. It is not easy to convey in a few words any idea of the ferment of activity in research, and much of it must in any case seem very remote from the daily tasks of those coping with MS and its many problems. I do not know when a cure or effective prevention will be discovered but these are now the objectives of many powerful research teams and I trust and believe that success will not be long delayed.

Index

Collin

061 294 2060

SHITT/ 756104/ A99EH.

97·00 .